Health Policy

Health Policy

A Critical Perspective

Iain Crinson

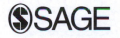

Los Angeles • London • New Delhi • Singapore • Washington DC

SAGE Publications Ltd
1 Oliver's Yard
55 City Road
London EC1Y 1SP

SAGE Publications Inc.
2455 Teller Road
Thousand Oaks, California 91320

SAGE Publications India Pvt Ltd
B 1/I 1 Mohan Cooperative Industrial Area
Mathura Road
New Delhi 11 044

SAGE Publications Asia-Pacific Pte Ltd
33 Pekin Street #02-01
Far East Square
Singapore 048763

Library of Congress Control Number: 2008928384

British Library Cataloguing in Publication data

A catalogue record for this book is available from
the British Library

ISBN 978-1-4129-2286-9
ISBN 978-1-4129-2287-6(pbk)

Typeset by CEPHA Imaging Pvt Ltd, Bangalore, India
Printed in Great Britain by TJ International Ltd, Padstow, Cornwall
Printed on paper from sustainable resources

Mixed Sources
Product group from well-managed
forests and other controlled sources
www.fsc.org   Cert no. SGS-COC-2482
FSC   © 1996 Forest Stewardship Council

CONTENTS

ACKNOWLEDGEMENTS

Every effort has been made to trace all the copyright holders, but if any have been inadvertently overlooked the publishers will be pleased to make the necessary arrangement at the first opportunity. I would like to dedicate this book to my children, Elliott and Miles, and to Lorna who has given me invaluable support and motivation to undertake and complete this text.

INTRODUCTION

For over two decades now, the structure and organisation of healthcare in Britain has been in a permanent state of transformation and change. The Conservative government under Margaret Thatcher's leadership initiated this period of reform by seeking to introduce market forces into the post-war state system of healthcare. The New Labour government which came into power in 1997 was in principle committed to reversing many of these policies and to a return to the founding principles of the NHS. In practice, the New Labour government has been more reform-orientated than the previous government. An almost continuous stream of policy initiatives has emerged over the last decade, designed to meet the government's political goal of retaining healthcare as a public service whilst offering patients more choice through the development of a 'supplier market' in healthcare provision.

But how do we make sense of these constant shifts in health policy? Should the public pronouncements of health ministers be accepted at face value? Or should health policy be seen purely as a pragmatic response by government to changing political demands without any long-term strategic plan? Can a broader set of social, political and organisational processes which have shaped policy development be identified? There is certainly a need for a much more integrated and theoretical perspective in health policy textbooks in order to contextualise what often amounts to a rather superficial and chronological account of a series of government policy initiatives.

Policy studies have traditionally eschewed explicit theorisation (although it has always been present implicitly) reflecting its origins in social administration, but this can have the consequence of providing students with a sea of information with no map to guide their journey through the complexities of health policy. The aim of this textbook is to integrate conceptual themes drawn from sociology and political science in analysing health policy. The focus on conceptual linkages will demonstrate the continuities in policy practice, and avoid the impression of newness or innovation that governments like to convey. The aim being to contextualise 'the reforms' in the healthcare system within a wider understanding of social and political processes in order to avoid descriptive and historicist accounts of health policy formation.

Michael Hill (1997) has identified four possible approaches to the study and analysis of social and health policy :

(a) Analysis *of* policy – with the aim of furthering an understanding of specific policy
(b) Analysis *for* policy – with the aim of improving the quality of policy
(c) Analysis concerned with *ends* – evaluating the outcome of a policy
(d) A concern with *means* – the policy process

This book will adopt all four approaches. Additionally, it is hoped that as students develop a critical understanding of the policy process they themselves will be able to influence and participate in both process and policy advocacy in the field of healthcare.

THE STRUCTURE

The first section of the book is concerned with theoretically contextualising the study of contemporary health policy. The first chapter begins by examining the field of health policy studies. Where there was once a broad agreement about the main constituents of the study of health policy, today many of these assumptions are being challenged and subject to dispute. In introducing the reader to the field of health policy studies, this chapter examines the range of theoretical frameworks that are drawn upon in the contemporary analyses of policy, and includes a discussion of power as a key analytical concept. The second chapter builds on these conceptualisations of power in order to examine the nature of state power in modern societies in the context of its role as the major provider (and purchaser) of healthcare in Britain. The major conceptualisations of the role played by the modern state in democratic societies are outlined, and the theoretical and philosophical differences that exist between them are identified. The final chapter in this section of the book analyses the process of making policy. The formal and informal processes involved in the formation, development, implementation and assessment of health policy initiatives are examined in the context of the NHS being one of the largest bureaucratic organisations in Western Europe. The issue of whether the political processes involved in policy-making are purely a 'reactive' pragmatic response to some emergent set of social and health problems, or whether a defined and distinct set of political ideas and values shape policy is explored.

The second section of the book examines the constituents of what are termed healthcare 'systems'. The first chapter in this section examines the organisational structure of healthcare in the UK, and assesses the organisational transitions that have occurred throughout the sixty year history of the NHS. The second chapter in this section examines the sources of funding of the NHS, the issue of 'under-funding', and goes on to critically assesses the expanding role of private finance in the state healthcare system. The third chapter in the section provides a comparative analysis of European national healthcare systems. This analysis is presented as a method of avoiding the pitfalls of studying the UK healthcare system in isolation, which can lead to a over- or underestimation of the uniqueness of the problems faced by the NHS. The key learning objective of the chapter for readers to appreciate that the health policy responses of other European Union countries address a common set of concerns around delivery of healthcare and meeting health needs.

The third section of the book focuses on specific issues in contemporary healthcare policy and provision. It seeks to provide a historical background and organisational context to a detailed examination of New Labour health policy. The first chapter in this section looks at the role played by the medical profession in the structuring of the NHS, who as 'gatekeepers' to the service were able to determine health need and set priorities for healthcare spending. Over the last twenty years, central government has sought to re-establish its control over the activities of the medical profession through a series of organisational developments designed to extend managerial control over the autonomy and self-regulation traditionally enjoyed by doctors. The second chapter examines the management and performance of the NHS. New internal regulatory systems and performance assessment frameworks have been established over the past two decades with the goal of improving the organisational performance of the NHS. The chapter examines the ways in which these managerialist solutions can become derailed by organisational cultures resistant to change. The third chapter explores the development of the 'Patient-led NHS'. This is a vision of the NHS in which users are given a greater range of choices about who will provide the care they require. This process is being facilitated by the construction of a new supplier market in which service provision is commissioned from a range of healthcare providers from the public, private and voluntary sectors. This chapter draws upon a critical conceptualisation of consumerism in order to assess the thinking behind these recent reforms, and whether equity of access to NHS services is narrowing rather than widening as a consequence of this shift in policy. The final chapter in this section examines how the increasing demand for long-term care in the community has brought about a fundamental reform of health and social care services. This chapter sets out a conceptualisation of 'social needs', and then looks at the way in which such needs are now assessed by the state and the logic behind the imposition of new eligibility criteria for care. The chapter goes on to critically assess some of the assumptions of policy makers about the role of families, and particularly of women, in providing care and support for those with long-term health and social care needs.

The final section of the book assesses the increasingly limited ability of health policies to limit or reduce threats to the health of the population. It examines the processes by which governments were able to ignore the widening of social inequalities in the UK, and the challenges faced by the new Labour government in reducing this gap in health outcomes between social groups. The chapter also analyses the development of the strategy of health promotion associated with the changing nature of the relationship of governance between state and citizen in managing or preventing health risks. The chapter concludes by looking at the increasing globalised nature of health risks which can affect the health of all.

USING THIS BOOK

This text utilises a series of case studies to illustrate how health policies have been implemented in practice. These are designed to show the importance of the social and organisational context in which top-down policy is enacted. A series of what are termed 'Key Concepts' appear throughout the text: these are designed to introduce the reader to the relevance of theory in assessing the formation and implementation of health policy. Also present throughout the text are a number of activities that enable readers to develop their understanding of the issues discussed in the text. These activities include references to further sources of information that the reader can utilise in completing the activity.

PART ONE

THEORY AND CONTEXT

1   STUDYING HEALTH POLICY

INTRODUCTION

Where there was once a broad agreement about the main constituents of the study of health policy, many of these assumptions are today subject to dispute. In introducing the reader to the field of health policy studies, this chapter examines the divergent theoretical frameworks that are drawn upon in the contemporary analyses of policy and, in particular, the differences in the way in which political power is conceptualised.

WHAT IS A 'POLICY'?

Policy as a concept is neither a specific, nor indeed a concrete phenomenon, so to attempt to define it poses a number of problems. It is more fruitful to see policy as a course of action or '*web of decisions*' or decision network, rather than a single identifiable decision (Hill, 1997: 7). Policies are on-going and dynamic and therefore are subject to change, particularly in response to problems arising out of implementation of a decision. Policy can also be just as much about inaction ('non-decision-making') as action; the maintenance of the status quo. Policy can also be an outcome of actions taken over a period of time, by 'low-level actors' within an organisation, which have not been formally sanctioned by a decision taken by those at the 'top level'. Here, policy can be seen as emerging as the outcome of a set of processes rather than as a formal decision to follow a course of action. It should also be noted that in the French language no distinction is made between the words 'policy' and 'politics'. In this sense, a formal model of policy-making would be rejected in favour of an understanding of 'policy' as political in the widest sense of the word.

DEFINING THE CHARACTERISTICS OF PUBLIC POLICY

Is there then anything distinctive about public policy as against those policies adopted by corporate organisations or even those of individuals? In terms of simple characteristics, the answer is 'no'. However, because public or state policy emanates from the government as the legal authority within a society nation, it follows that it has a primacy and influence over all other policies (private and personal). These public policies provide the legalistic framework through which individuals must operate. A private company for example cannot decide that it wants to employ women at a lower rate of pay for performing a job than male employees doing the same job. This is because it would be in breach of the Equal Opportunities legislation and therefore subject to legal sanctions.

One possible starting point in attempting to define public policy and policy-making is to examine how the UK government itself has presented these issues. Relatively early on in its first term in office, the New Labour government published a White Paper entitled *Modernising Government* (Cabinet Office, 1999), which sets out the 'official' view of policy-making as follows: 'Policy making is the process by which governments translate their political vision into programmes and actions to deliver "outcomes" – desired changes in the real world' (Cabinet Office, 1999: para 2.1). The White Paper goes on to outline the six key characteristics associated with what it termed a 'modernising' (health, social, economic, etc.) policy; these characteristics are set out below:

- *Strategic* – A modernising policy looks ahead and contributes to long-term government goals.
- *Outcome focused* – A modernising policy aims to deliver desired changes in the real world.
- *Joined up* – A modernising policy operates across the organisational boundaries of government.
- *Inclusive* – A modernising policy is fair and takes account of the interests of all.
- *Flexible and Innovative* – A modernising policy tackles cause, not symptoms, and is not afraid of experimentation.

- *Robust* – A modernising policy stands the test of time and works in practice from the start.

This definition will be returned to again later within the book as one possible outcome measure of health policy, utilising the government's own terms of reference.

SCOPING THE FIELD OF HEALTH POLICY ANALYSIS

The academic study of health policy in the UK has traditionally been focused upon the formal institutions of the welfare state charged with the treatment and care of the sick. The primary concern of these studies has been the analysis of the organisations and structure of the NHS, as well as the rather more poorly defined area of public health. From the late 1950s onwards, health and social policy studies as an academic discipline established a conceptual base, drawing almost exclusively upon its own internal theoretical and analytical frameworks, rooted in a set of implicit political and philosophical assumptions associated with the emergence and development of the post-war welfare state. This *de facto* delineation of the academic study of health policy effectively played down the potential contribution of the disciplines of sociology, politics and economics to policy analysis. However, over the last two decades this rather narrow approach to the subject has come under sustained criticism, largely as a consequence of real world political developments. The health and social policies of the Conservative governments of the late 1980s and early 1990s, and to a debatable extent those of the New Labour governments since 1997, have sustained the neo-liberal challenge to the very idea of universal state provision of social welfare and health services. Thus, the very basis of an academic discipline centred on the welfare state was itself disrupted. It was now no longer appropriate or relevant to study social and health policy in isolation from other forms of social organisation and social structures (Coffey, 2004: 3).

The work of many of the early pioneers of health and social policy analysis in Britain, such as that of Richard Titmuss (1958, 1970), Peter Townsend (1970a), and Brian Abel-Smith (Abel-Smith and Townsend, 1966), was informed by a detailed sociological analysis of the workings of the welfare state and its impact on the health and social welfare services on the lives of ordinary people. These studies revealed that the health and welfare needs of many of the most deprived groups in post-war Britain were not being met because the state left the forces of the market economy largely unchecked. These structures of exploitation were seen to reproduce poverty across the generations and to sustain poor levels of health. The criticisms levelled at the academic discipline of health and social policy analysis in the 1980s and 1990s were that it chose to focus on organisational matters whilst all too often it neglected to assess whether the founding social and political goals of the welfare state (including the NHS) were still relevant to the health and social needs of the population – for example, whether the worst effects of poverty and low income were being addressed, or whether access to good quality healthcare was available to all irrespective of social status and income. These were the original concerns that inspired the work of Titmuss, Townsend and Abel-Smith, who, whilst supportive of the goals of the welfare state, always engaged in a critical analysis of the practice of the NHS and other state welfare institutions.

As will be apparent from the discussion in the introductory chapter, the aim of this book is to engage in a process of critical analysis of contemporary health policy. The first stage in this process, given the previous discussion concerning the limitations of traditional analytical approaches, is to delineate in its widest sense the potential field of health policy analysis. This means moving beyond the confines of an analysis of the formal institutions of healthcare, and assessing all those policies (both public and private) that impact upon health and well-being of the population, employing the conceptual tools of both sociology and political science; this scope of policy analysis is set out in Figure 1.1.

THE FORMAL HEALTHCARE SYSTEM

This was gradually constructed over the course of a century-and-a-half in order to better manage the clinical needs of those in the population who were sick and disabled, and this largely remains its focus to this day. The healthcare system in Britain has historically never given priority to disease prevention and health promotion. Apart from policies directly affecting the formal healthcare system itself, also included in Figure 1.1 are the following areas with potential impacts on the health outcomes of the population, and which therefore should be a concern of health policy analysis.

ENVIRONMENTAL PROTECTION

This covers areas such as atmospheric pollution, the use of toxic chemicals and radiation, the effects of global warming, the use of non-renewable resources, the planting of genetically modified (GM) crops, and many other developments with the potential to compromise the natural environment and therefore negatively affect the long-term health of the population. Policies include the attempt to reduce carbon emissions, the promotion of renewable energy sources and recycling, and the safeguarding of individuals from the effects of poor air quality.

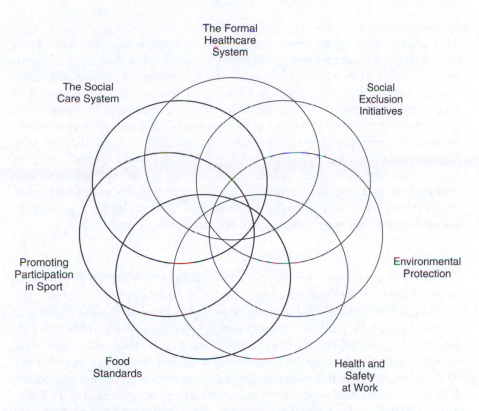

Figure 1.1 Scoping the field of health policy analysis

FOOD STANDARDS

This is the area of state regulation and enforcement of legislation which serves to protect the public's health and consumer interests in relation to food. This covers issues of food hygiene, nutritional standards, and food labelling.

HEALTH AND SAFETY AT WORK

The Health and Safety Commission (HSC) and the Health and Safety Executive (HSE) are responsible for the enforcement of legislation and the regulation of almost all the risks to health and safety arising from work activity in Britain, as well as many other aspects of the protection both of workers and the public.

SOCIAL CARE SYSTEM

This covers those aspects of care provided or purchased by local authorities outside the formal healthcare system for those living with chronic illness and disability, learning and physical disabilities, as well as those with long-term mental health problems.

SOCIAL EXCLUSION INITIATIVES

This covers those government intervention programmes that have been introduced over the past decade in order to remove families from living in poverty, with all its negative impact on long-term health. These initiatives include the *Sure Start* programme, designed to improve the health and emotional development for young children living in deprived communities by increasing the availability of childcare for all children and supporting parents in their aspirations towards employment. Britain also has the highest rate of teenage pregnancy of any Western European country. This 'social problem' is seen to reflect low expectations as well as economic deprivation, and as such is recognised as having long-term health and social implications for both the young mothers and their children; a nationally coordinated action plan now aims to reduce this high rate.

PROMOTING PARTICIPATION IN SPORT

It has become a truism that the popularity of sport in Britain is restricted to watching it rather than active participation. *Sport England* (formerly the English Sports Council) is the body responsible for distributing funds and providing strategic guidance for promoting sporting activity in England. Its slogan is 'Get active, healthy and happy', which emphasises the importance of sport participation for the health of a largely sedentary population. The funding for this organisation comes from central government and the National Lottery, and since 1994, it has invested over £2bn of Lottery funds and £300 million from the Treasury into supporting not only professional sport but in promoting greater community participation in sport in England. However, with the awarding of the 2012 Olympic Games to London, the debate about whether disproportionate amounts of public money is spent on elite rather than grassroots sport has widened.

All those areas where policy impacts upon health outcome will be explored in the book, although the substantive focus will be upon the formal healthcare system. However, the analysis will not be restricted to an examination of White Papers, strategy documents and the top-down interventions by the Department of Health. A significant concern of this textbook is how these centrally devised policies are interpreted and implemented in practice.

CONCEPTUAL FRAMEWORKS IN THE ANALYSIS OF HEALTH POLICY

Having delineated the field of health policy analysis the next stage is to critically examine the range of conceptual frameworks that are used to assess health policy.

All academic and indeed all so-called common-sense understanding, whether practical or theoretical, involves the use of some sort of model or conceptual schema in order to simplify and make sense of the tremendous variety of potential variables that exist in the social and physical world. In the complex process of health policy formation and implementation within a dynamic political and economic system such as exists within the UK, the application of conceptual frameworks is essential if we are to gain an understanding of the hows and whys of current health policy. These frameworks are drawn from a variety of often conflicting theoretical perspectives. For example, the analysis of the institutions and organisational processes associated with the modern welfare state has traditionally been heavily reliant upon models which derive from a theorisation of the historical role of the State as vehicle for the social and national transformation and development. However, this is just one theorisation of the role of the State within modern capitalist societies, there are many other competing explanations of the role of the State that can be found within sociological analysis; these are discussed in detail in Chapter 2.

As discussed in the Introduction, the aim of this textbook is to contextualise the essentially political process of formulating and implementing health policy by locating specific developments within a broader set of social and institutional processes. This involves synthesising theoretical constructs relevant to the analysis with an empirical description of the specific processes associated with the development of a particular policy. This is what is meant by integrating theory with practice. Hence, while the opening chapters of the book give broad descriptions of the range of theoretical frameworks utilized within policy analysis, this should not be seen as a process of 'front-loading'. Where they are most relevant to the discussion of specific health policy developments, 'key concepts' deriving from a wide range of theoretical traditions within sociology and political theory will be introduced to facilitate analysis. This approach is designed to avoid a tendency which is sometimes found in policy analysis, which acknowledges the importance of theory whilst failing to explicitly integrate it in practice.

At a general analytical level, health policy can be conceptualised in terms of macro and micro social processes. At a macro level this involves the assessment of the workings of social and institutional structures such as the State, the market, economic and legal frameworks, as well as formal institutions of social welfare such as the NHS. At a micro level of analysis, the focus is on the impact of policy at the level of the practice of healthcare professionals, as well as upon the experiences of the users of the service as they negotiate their way through the often labyrinthine pathways of the State healthcare system.

'POWER' AS A KEY CONCEPT FOR CRITICAL HEALTH POLICY ANALYSIS

This first chapter concludes with an outline of 'power', an essential conceptual tool in any critical analysis of the formation and implementation of health policy. Following this outline you are invited to participate in an exercise which assesses your understanding of power by exploring the idea that a health policy need not necessarily be about innovation and change but can also be about maintaining the status quo.

The notion of 'power' is very much a contested construct, and its use in policy analysis is therefore highly value-dependent. Conceptualisations of power reflect particular moral and political positions, and usually rest on normatively specific conception of interests (Lukes, 1974). So, for example, the Cabinet Office (1999) definition of policy sees it as the ability, '... to deliver outcomes – desired changes in the real world'. This definition carries with it an implicit conceptualisation of power as something deriving from the democratic mandate of an elected government charged with instigating a programme of policy reform. While the classic presentation of power within social theory is that it represents, '... the chance of a man or a number of men to realize their own will in a communal action even against the resistance of others who are participating in the action' (Weber, 1978: 926).

This definition raises the question of whether in the absence of any observable conflict, power is actually being exercised. This issue was explored in Dahl's influential work in which he argued that power resides in the *potential* a person has to influence and direct the behaviour of others; reflected in the much quoted position that, '*A* has power over *B* to the extent that he can get *B* to do something that *B* would not otherwise do' (Dahl, 1957). This is a conceptualisation of power as a form of domination, manifested in successful acts of decision-making. However, this view of power has been criticised as being overly narrow and conceived primarily in relational terms. Lukes (2004) has argued that whilst the empirical observation of the exercise of power in decision-making can provide evidence of its possession, and that the counting of 'power resources' such as wealth, status and influence can provide evidence of how power is distributed within a given society, power is primarily, '... a *capacity* and not the exercise or the vehicle of that capacity' (2004: 70). Power is seen as a potentiality rather than an actuality, in that it does not need to be seen to be exercised to exist.

In his seminal work written in the 1970s, Lukes (1974; 2004) identified three 'dimensions' of power. What he termed the 'one-dimensional view' is the Weberian conceptualisation that is described above. It is one-dimensional because it is seen to focus exclusively on observable behaviour (reflecting Weber's primary concern with social action rather than structures) in the making of conscious decisions around an identified controversial issue. While this view of power offers a relatively straightforward pathway for policy studies because of its focus on the decision-making of key political agents, for Lukes it is essentially blind to the ways in which the policy agenda is controlled (1974: 58). The 'two-dimensional view' is one in which power is conceived of as involving both decision-making and non-decision-making. Where a decision is defined as a choice among alternative 'modes of action', and a non-decision is one that results in 'suppression or thwarting' of either a 'latent or manifest challenge' to the interests of the decision-maker (1974: 44). Those with power exercise it to prevent particular issues being placed on the policy agenda or to prevent decisions being taken. Thus, in policy analysis it becomes important to examine not just issues about which observable political decisions are made, but also to identify potential issues which non-decision-making prevents from being actual issues for political debate.

Lukes's (1974) critique of this two-dimensional view is that while it attempts to move beyond an exclusive focus on actual decision-making behaviour, it nevertheless continues to place too much emphasis on the actions of individuals within that system. Lukes argues that attention should also be given to the ways in which these actions arise from the socially structured and culturally patterned behaviour of groups of decision-makers (1974: 22). Both the one- and the two-dimensional views presuppose that power is only exercised in situations of actual conflict between different interest groups, but this position often fails to acknowledge that, '... the most effective and insidious use of power is to prevent such conflict from arising in the first place' (1974: 23). Lukes goes on to argue that it is a mistake to assume that non-decision-making power, '... only exists where there are grievances which are denied entry into the political process in the form of issues' (1974: 24). This ignores the possibility that the interests of social groups have not already been shaped so that they '... accept their role in the existing order of things, either because they can see or imagine no alternative to it, or because they see it as natural and unchangeable' (1974: 24).

Lukes argues that it is therefore necessary to think in terms of a third dimension in which the exercise of power is constituted in the ability to manipulate and shape the wants, needs, values and norms of behaviour of a population. This is achieved through the hegemony (or leadership) of a dominant group in a society, exercising power through ideological structures such as the education system, the media, and various other socialisation processes. Thus, in the political policy-making process there is both observable conflict (the first and second dimensions) and latent conflict arising out of the contradictions between the interests of those exercising power and the 'real interests' of those they exclude (1974: 25).

An alternative and highly influential reading of power is present in the work of Michel Foucault (1979a; 1980) who sought to 're-conceptualise' power by seeing it not as a property of individual or collective social agents, but as 'a machine that no one owns'. That is, as society has transformed itself into its modern form so power became 'knowledge', in that objects and events are interpreted or constituted using knowledge not only in theoretical terms but in everyday practice. A unity of thought in a particular society at a particular time constitutes what is seen to be rational or 'the truth of a situation', and therefore valid and worthy of discussion. This form of power has the effect of excluding other explanations.

ACTIVITY

(a) Identify an issue which you perceive as negatively affecting your own health and that of your family in some way. The issue can be as broad or as narrow as you like. For example, it could be that you would like your child's school to provide healthy options rather than processed food for school lunch; you want the government to take more proactive steps to reduce environmental pollution; your employers refuse to take steps to reduce the amount of stress that you experience at work; etc.

(b) Then identify with reasons for your decision which of the theorisations of the nature of power described above (Weber's decision-making process model, Lukes' third dimension, or Foucault's discursive practices) that you think best explains the failure to act upon the problematic health issue that you have identified?

ACTIVITY 1 – COMMENTARY

Whatever health issue you have identified, it is likely to be one that you regard as being beyond your individual ability to change. This may have led you on to the question of who or what (a political figure, a local institution or central government) has the power to bring about such change. Questions may have also arisen such as: Who do I approach in order to present my grievance?; Is there a formal public accountability system in place to allow me to present the issues? Or whether you perceive the system to be intractable and unresponsive to your needs? If the latter is the case, do you think that some form of extra-institutional pressure can be brought to bear on the key decision-makers through some form of collective action through the means of tenants associations, trade unions, or parents/patients groups?

SUMMARY

This chapter has introduced students to the field of health policy and raised the issue of the importance of appreciating the importance of the conceptual framework that is employed in the analysis of the policy process. The political, moral and philosophical assumptions underpinning this framework will therefore shape the form of the analysis. The contested nature of power as a key conceptualisation employed in health and social policy analysis was also highlighted as a preliminary to the detailed assessment of the construction of health policy in later chapters.

FURTHER READING

Hill, M. (2004) *The Public Policy Process*, (4th Edn). Harlow: Pearson Longman.

Clarke, J. (2004) *Changing Welfare, Changing States: New Directions in Social Policy*. London: Sage.

Lukes, S. (2004) *Power: A Radical View*, (2nd Edn). London: Palgrave.

2 THE ROLE OF THE STATE: THEORY AND PRACTICE

CHAPTER CONTENTS

- Introduction
- Theorising the modern state
- Case study: Adopting a path-dependency approach in comparing British health policy in the 1950s with that of the 1980s
- Conceptualising the role of the welfare state in healthcare provision
- Summary

INTRODUCTION

Building on the general theories of power explored in the previous chapter, the primary concern of this chapter is to examine the nature of state power in modern societies in the context of its role as the major provider and purchaser of healthcare in the UK. The theoretical and philosophical differences that exist between theories of the state are identified. These competing theorisations are then assessed in relation to the efficacy of the analysis of the state provision of health and welfare services within the UK. The chapter concludes with a brief outline of the debate concerning the direction of state health and welfare provision in the twenty-first century. Are we witnessing an expansion of the regulatory role of the state in shaping the structure of health services for its citizens, or are we seeing the emergence of a deregulated state in which the private market plays a much greater role in meeting the healthcare choices of 'consumers' of the health services?

Theorisations of the role of the state range from those which see it as being an essentially neutral instrument enacting the will of the people in a participatory democratic system, whilst others see the state as acting primarily to maintain the social and economic interests of powerful groups within society. Important distinctions also exist in the way in which the health and welfare role of the state is historically, socially, and politically contextualised. This chapter is not intended as a definitive theoretical assessment of the modern capitalist state and its health and welfare role, rather the intention is to sign-post a key theme of this text, that of the contested nature of state health and welfare policy. This is a view endorsed by David Held when he asserted that, '(T)here is nothing more central to political and social theory than the nature of the state, and nothing more contested' (Held, 1983: 1).

THEORISING THE MODERN STATE

In attempting to define the role of the modern state Christopher Pierson has written that:

> We might find it difficult to give a precise and comprehensive definition of the state, but we think we recognize it when it flags us down on the motorway, sends us a final tax demand or, of course, arranges for our old age pension to be paid at the nearest post office ... everyday political discussion is replete with appeals to, condemnation of and murmurings about the state (Pierson, 1996: 5).

There exist a wide range of theorisations of the role of the state in modern societies; six of the most influential conceptualisations are compared in Figure 2.1, which utilises a matrix in order to assess their differences and commonalities along two key dimensions. Firstly, in terms of whether the models see the state as a 'neutral instrument' carrying out the requirements of a society (termed 'society-centred'), or whether the state is conceived as having an independent or autonomous role in shaping the organisation

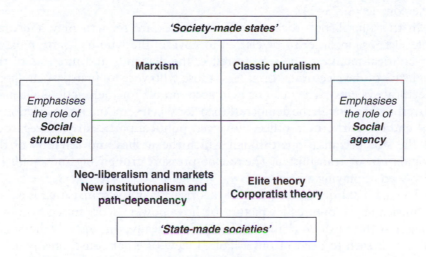

Figure 2.1   A four dimensional matrix of the major theorisations of the modern state

and structure of a society; following Pierson (1996: 70) this pole of the dimension is termed 'state-made societies'. The second dimension of the matrix draws attention to the other major distinction found within state theory, the relative degree of power attributed to social agency (the activities of individuals and social groups in pursuance of their interests) as against social structure (economic and political forces shaping activities of social agents) in determining the shape and role of the modern state within a society.

Having identified where this range of theories of the state sit in relation to two key dimensions, each model will now be described in outline, beginning with those theories of the state that emphasise the role of social agency.

CLASSIC PLURALISM

The primary assumption of this model is that modern democratic political states, such as exist in Britain and the USA, serve to represent the plurality and diversity of these societies. Power within these societies, following Parsons (1951), is seen as something possessed by society as a whole and is the capacity to mobilise the resources of a given society in order to achieve the political goals democratically voted on by the electorate. Whilst not denying the existence of social divisions such as class, gender, ethnicity, classic pluralists would reject the view that any one of these social divisions exclusively influences any particular individual's wishes or actions; each of us having many different possibly competing interests. Public policy outcomes are therefore reflective of the balance of forces and social divisions in society registered, but not mediated, by government in the 'public interest' (Pierson, 1996: 73–74).

In this pluralistic process, political parties are seen to play a pivotal role, because in order to be elected to govern, the winning party must in its political manifesto be seen to reflect the demands and interests of the majority of the electorate (or at least those who vote in 'first-past-the-post' electoral systems). They can be held accountable for their actions when in government through the democratic process when standing for re-election at the end of their term in office. However, political parties are not regarded as the sole organisations through which the wishes and interests of the population are transmitted. The role of 'pressure groups' big and small, are also seen as playing a role.

The main critique of the pluralist theorisation of the state is that it paints a 'misleadingly optimistic' picture of how power is organised within a society such as Britain (Hill, 1997: 34). Specifically, this view of the policy process is seen to derive from a limited view of what constitutes political power as it focuses only upon the observable exercise of power. While most modern pluralists would acknowledge that power is not equally distributed, they would nevertheless see the political system as equally open to all and reject Weber's concept of power as a 'constant-sum', a fixed amount held by one group at the expense of others.

THEORIES OF ELITES

Elite theory, was first represented in the work of Mosca (1939) who recognised that a ruling minority will always exist in societies because of the unequal distribution of wealth, talent and intellect. So, although democratically elected governments formally represent the 'will of the people', these governments are constituted by elites with their own sets of interests. In its classic form, elite theory sees a variety of social elites who achieve their position of power in a political system by virtue of their control over key resources. In modern societies this is invariably control over economic resources, but can also include knowledge and expertise, as well as being based on traditional forms of high social status. Weber (1963) recognised the existence of a 'circulation of elites' holding political power and able to direct the actions of a large scale bureaucracy (Weber's work on the emergence of modern bureaucratic forms of the state is described in detail in Chapter 3). As Schumpeter famously stated it, '(D)emocracy does not mean and cannot mean that the people actually rule in any obvious sense of the terms "people" and "rule". Democracy means only that the people have the opportunity of accepting or refusing the men who are to rule them ...' (Schumpeter, 1976: 284).

A more radical and critical theory of elitism is present in the work of C. Wright Mills (1956). Writing in the America of the 1950s, Mills argued that certain institutions (the military, major industrial corporations, and the US government) held 'pivotal positions' in society. The individuals holding the top positions within these institutions were seen to have similar sets of interests and mutually supported each other, forming a 'national power elite'. Today, in countries like Britain, many would recognise the existence of such a political power elite which would include government ministers, executives of large multi-national corporations, senior judges, top civil servants and heads of NGOs; although this would be a rather more fragmented social group than was suggested in the C.W. Mills model.

Another form of elitist theory, known as corporatist theory, argues that the state is forced into a more interventionist role when national economic growth slows down as a consequence of international competition. The state is seen to act as a powerful intermediary, bringing together major organised business and labour interests in order to encourage the development of collaborative policies for growth. This process occurred to a greater or lesser extent in Britain between 1950 to 1979, and remains the formal model influencing the role of the state in Germany, Sweden and France.

The issue though, is whether corporatist theory is seen as an ideal model of government, or whether it actually represents an over-estimate of the power the state bureaucracy has to effect change and direct the structuring of the economy and business (Pierson, 1996: 88).

A general critique of elitist theories is that they do not fundamentally diverge from pluralist models in that most recognise a circulation of social elites rather than a fixed ruling class. With the possible exception of Wright Mills, elite theories also share with pluralist models a disregard for the question of how elites acquire and hold on to power; these are the structural questions which are emphasised in the alternate models of the state discussed below.

The second part of this section examines those theories of the state that emphasise the determining role of structure. Whilst these theories embrace widely divergent views on just how determinist these structural forces are within a given society, what they do have in common is a recognition that the state policy process is strongly influenced by powerful forces outside of individual or group control. However, it should be said that most structuralist theories do acknowledge that structure is not completely deterministic and that social agency plays some part in shaping the role of state.

MARXIST APPROACHES

Marx's own analysis begins with an understanding of the pivotal role played by the material base of a given society, the demands of the system of economic production. In the capitalist system of economic production, Marx sees the modern state as essentially an instrument of the ruling capitalist class. However, in certain of his writings he also recognised that in particular sets of circumstances the state could exert a degree of independence or 'relative autonomy' from this capitalist class. This enabled the state to 'appear to stand above society' in order to better exercise its power to maintain social cohesion and the long-term conditions for capital accumulation.

Since the 1960s, Marxist theories of the state have developed in a number of directions, but most distance themselves from a purely instrumental understanding of the role of the state as being directly controlled by the capitalist class. This in large part reflects the enduring influence of Antonio Gramsci (1971), who, whilst a prisoner of Mussolini's fascist Italian government in the 1930s, set out a new perspective of the state and society relationship. Gramsci argued that in the 'advanced' form of capitalism that was being developed in the West in the interwar period, the rule of the capitalist class could not be secured primarily through state repression and control. In everyday interaction, the interests of capitalist production were seen to be maintained through the institutions of 'civil society', such as the church, media, the educational system and other forms of cultural practices, rather than through the more coercive apparatuses of the state such as the law or armed forces. Gramsci was particularly interested in those ideological and political practices which interweaved the actions of the state and the institutions of civil society in maintaining the legitimacy and 'hegemony' (or dominance) of the ruling class, resulting in the population giving their 'active consent' to their own economic exploitation (The key concepts of ideology and hegemony are outlined below). This is then a broad and all-inclusive conception of the state, which goes beyond an analysis of the legislature (i.e., Parliament) and executive structures of government to embrace all the political, ideological and cultural structures ('apparatuses') through which social cohesion is maintained.

KEY CONCEPT – IDEOLOGY & HEGEMONY

Ideology as a theoretical construct has been subject to many conflicting uses within social theory:

> … (it) has been utilised to designate anything from a contemplative attitude that misrecognises its dependence on social reality to an action-orientated set of beliefs, from the indispensable medium in which individuals live out their relations to a social structure to false ideas which legitimate a dominant political power (Zizék, 1989/1994: 4)

However, the range of meanings attached to the concept can be narrowed down to two quite distinct usages, reflecting two fundamentally different theoretical paradigms.

First, as used within political science, 'ideology' has come to denote a coherent system of political ideas (e.g., communism, liberalism, social democracy, etc.), and embraces sets of moral and ethical values, such as the meanings attached to ideas of social justice, equality, human needs and personal responsibilities; as well as more pragmatic political concerns. Second, as used within the social sciences, ideologies are understood in the broader sense of being discursive types of social phenomena, which can include the level of everyday notions and 'experience' as well as elaborate intellectual doctrines. Ideology can therefore be seen as operating not only at the level of the 'consciousness' of social actors but also at the level of institutionalised 'thought-systems' and discourses of a given society. Ideology operates to organise, maintain, reproduce and occasionally transform power within a society (Therborn, 1980: 2).

(Continued)

(*Continued*)

However, although ideas and values are very important in sustaining the dominance of particular groups and their self-interests, sometimes this is not enough and more structured and coercive methods are employed to achieve a political outcome. *Hegemony* is the term used to denote this domination or control of one group over another. Utilising the concept of hegemony in this context would include ideological processes, but would not be reducible to ideology.

Bob Jessop's (1990, 2002) influential 'strategic-relational' approach (SRA) is an example of a more recent Marxist-influenced structured approach which have abandoned Gramsci's 'relative autonomy' approach, replacing it with a view of the state as an 'operationally autonomous, institutionally separate political system'. Jessop defines the dynamic and complex set of social relations that he sees as characteristic of the modern state as, '(t)he relatively unified ensemble of socially embedded, socially regularized, and strategically selective institutions, organisations, social forces and activities, organised around making collectively binding decisions for an imagined political community'(2002: 40). The term 'strategically selective' refers to the ways in which the state has a 'specific and differential' impact on the ability of competing political forces to pursue their particular interests and strategies. This process is seen as essentially a relational one because the ability to initiate a particular policy direction depends upon the relation between state structures and the strategies which various social forces adopt towards it (Jessop, 1990: 10). The strategic-relational approach is an assertion of the contingency and indeterminacy of social and political change which characterises the role of the state in capitalist societies, and which makes any definitive Marxist theory of the state highly elusive.

NEO-LIBERAL CONCEPTUALISATIONS OF THE STATE

A neo-liberal understanding of the role of state in health and welfare provision is one that combines explanation with prescription. The neo-liberal analysis perceives the state as 'an increasingly domineering and malign influence imposing itself upon society' (Pierson, 1996: 80). As a consequence, the leading polemicists of this approach, such as Milton Friedman (1962), advocated the promotion of the unimpeded 'free market' as the guarantee of liberty in modern societies because it established a separation between the social groups holding political power and those holding economic power. Another key figure in neo-liberal thought is Fredrich Hayek (1982) who argued that in those political systems where

Parliament is sovereign, governments become the plaything of organised sectional interests. In contradistinction to the pluralists he argued such interest group pressure is not the way in which the diversity of interest in society can be reconciled, rather it is the way in which organised groups promote their own interests at the expense of the general. For Hayek, these problems of unlimited government were exacerbated when social democratic governments with their social welfare/social justice political agenda were in power.

This neo-liberal approach asserts that collective choice exercised through state actions, beyond the absolute minimum safety net provisions, will always produce outcomes that are less efficient or desirable than outcomes determined by private choice in civil society delivered by means of the market (Pierson, 1996: 83). These views became part of the political mainstream when they were embraced in Britain by the Conservative Party in the mid-1970s, and in the same period by the Republican government in the USA.

NEW INSTITUTIONALISM

The thrust of this relatively new approach in social theory is to 'bring the state back into' the mainstream analysis of politics and society (Evans, Rueschemeyer and Skocpol, 1985). What those political theorists who hold to this view have in common is a critical view of the behaviour-orientated, social 'agent-centred' analysis of the role of the state (approaches which were particularly dominant in political science in the early 1980s), and the abandonment of the state as an analytical construct in favour of the more general notion of 'political systems'. The overriding concern is to argue that political decision-making processes cannot be understood without reference to the institutions in which these decisions occur. Schmidt (2006) has identified a number of forms of this 'new institutionalism' reflecting very different political, sociological and philosophical starting points. Each approach has a different object of explanation – such as the rational behaviour occurring within institutions, their historical structures, or their institutional norms and culture. Many of these approaches focus less on the role of the state itself, and more on the different kinds of action occurring within institutions of the state. Below, we will examine two of the more developed forms of new institutionalism, 'rational choice' and 'historical institutionalism'.

RATIONAL CHOICE INSTITUTIONALISM

Rational choice institutionalism theorises the state in terms of it being a rational actor pursuing a 'logic of interest', or as a structure of incentives within which rational policy actors follow their preferences. This approach developed from the need to seek a solution to the problems encountered by individual-orientated rational choice theory (which presents an ideal model of humankind who 'generate the entirety of the social structure from their inbuilt dispositions to be rational agents' Archer, 1998: 76), when attempting to predict the actual practice of policy-making. Bringing back an analysis of the institution itself was seen as a way of explaining the motivations and interests lying behind 'rational' political actors' behaviour within a given setting.

The main critique of this approach is that it analyses institutions largely in functional terms. That is, in relation to its effects or outcomes rather than in terms of the socio-economic and political processes that give rise to that state institution under analysis. Secondly, it is highly intentionalist because it assumes that rational actors are fully aware that they are the creations of and are controlled by the institution itself. Thirdly, because of its origins in rational choice theory it assumes fixed preferences for the policy actors based on an assumption of political stability, and therefore has difficulty in accounting for institutional change over time (Schmidt, 2006: 103).

HISTORICAL INSTITUTIONALISM

Unlike rational choice institutionalism, this approach explicitly focuses upon the development of the institution of the modern state (rather than its function alone). Its key assumption is that a historically constructed set of institutional constraints and opportunities influence the behaviour of politicians and interest groups involved in the policy-making process. According to Skocpol (1992), this approach views the domain of state politics ('the polity') as, '… the primary locus for action, yet understands political activities, whether carried by politicians or by social groups, as conditioned by institutional configurations of governments and party political systems' (1992: 41). This is a structural approach that recognises the autonomy of key political actors but is also able to acknowledge the influence of previously enacted policies on the decision-making of these actors. Schmidt has argued that historical institutionalism,

> … works best at delineating the origins and development of institutional structures and processes over time. It tends to focus on sequences in development, timing of events, and phases of political change. It emphasizes not just the asymmetries of power related to the operation and development of institutions but also the path-dependencies and unintended consequences that result from such historical development (Schmidt, 2006: 105).

Here, Schmidt draws particular attention to the concept of 'path-dependency', a construct now widely utilised in accounting for how state institutions develop over time, and which is described in detail below.

KEY CONCEPT – PATH-DEPENDENCY

Pierson (2000) has argued that path-dependence as a historical process has three distinct phases. First, where a particular event occurs within a sequence of events which can have disproportionately large effects later. Second, during the early stages of a sequence, a 'critical juncture' may occur in which the direction of policy gets more restrictive. Thirdly, as a policy pathway is followed, '… previously viable options may be foreclosed' as self-reinforcing feedback mechanisms encourage the move along one particular policy direction. Pierson (2000) identifies a number of these feedback mechanisms. One would be the incentive to continue in a particular direction because of the need to recoup the initial investment made by political actors (political parties, interest groups, bureaucracy) in a particular institution. Another would be 'learning effects'. This refers to the process whereby political actors operate within institutions that define a particular pathway become more adept and knowledgeable over time, and then use this to enhance the efficiency of that institution.

Mahoney has argued that path-dependence:

> characterizes those historical sequences in which contingent events set into motion institutional patterns or event chains that have deterministic properties. The identification of path-dependence therefore involves both tracing a given outcome back to a particular set of historical events, and showing how these events are themselves contingent occurrences that cannot be explained on the basis of prior historical conditions (Mahoney, 2000: 507–508).

Examples of the degree to which it is possible to discern a historical path-dependency within the National Health Service and the identification of feedback processes that operate within that institution that reinforce a particular direction in health policy will be explored throughout the text. One example of this approach to analysing the possible pathways through which state health policy is developed is set out below.

A CASE STUDY: ADOPTING A PATH-DEPENDENCY APPROACH IN COMPARING BRITISH HEALTH POLICY IN THE 1950s WITH THAT OF THE 1980s

This example of the theory of path-dependency draws on Ian Greener's (2001) study which emphasises the continuities found to be present within British government health policy vis-à-vis the NHS in the 1950s, and in the

1980s and 90s. In both cases, the Conservative Party came into power ideologically suspicious of the state health and welfare system it inherited, and committed to giving the private market a more substantive role in healthcare provision with the aim of reducing the tax burden on the electorate. This 'ideological and fiscal discomfort' manifested itself in both periods in an attempt to contain expenditure on the NHS in the face of rising demands on its services by patients, which led to a crisis of 'underfunding', and a search for alternative (non-Treasury) forms of funding for the service. However, as Greener notes, there were important '… structural barriers to implementing changes of this magnitude' (2001: 638).

Firstly, In both periods these attempts at reform were strongly opposed by the general public because of the considerable and enduring popularity of the NHS as an institution. The Conservative government, both in the 1950s and late 1980s, was highly vulnerable to the charge that it was dismantling the NHS through a process of 'privatisation'. Secondly, given the autonomy granted to the medical profession over the use of healthcare resources in the NHS (described in detail in Chapter 7), any reform of the organisation of healthcare required its support for successful implementation; and this was not achieved in both periods. As Greener argues, '(T)hese factors would seem to indicate that a degree of policy inertia tends to exist within the NHS and to confirm the view of path-dependent theorists of policy who would claim that structural forces dominate the policy process and that policy change is more likely to be incremental than paradigmatic' (2001: 638).

Greener concludes his study by arguing that, '… from time to time ideology might imply that the service should be radically reformed, but it remains recognizable from its 1948 incarnation. To employ an overused term, we are still within the same healthcare paradigm; still grappling with many of the problems first highlighted by commentators in the 1950s' (Greener, 2001: 643). However, whatever the apparent similarities between the problems faced by policy-makers in the 1950s and 1980s that this use of path-dependency approach draws attention to, the study can be criticised on the grounds that it underplays the differences between the demands on the NHS in the 1950s and in the 1980s and 1990s. One of the main differences is the pressure to meet the healthcare needs of an increasing proportion of elderly people in the population, which required the Conservative government of the early 1990s to increase public funding of primary care as well as community-based social care services. This shift in turn enabled the private market to become increasingly entrenched in service provision – a process that has continued under the New Labour government. This shift reflected a break rather than a continuity with the hitherto dominance of the hospital as the arena of healthcare provision dominated by the biomedical model of healthcare provision.

CONCEPTUALISING THE ROLE OF THE WELFARE STATE IN HEALTHCARE PROVISION

The evolution of the role of the British state as public provider of health and welfare services is subject to considerable debate and difference in the social and health policy literature. Five distinct conceptualisations of this role can identified (see Table 2.1). The differences between these conceptualisations reflect not only the range of assumptions found within state theory discussed above, they also reflect differences between political and ideological prescriptions of the role that the state *should* play in the provision and delivery of health and welfare services. For example, the neo-liberal perspective strongly influenced the shift in the health and welfare policies of the Conservative governments led by Margaret Thatcher in the 1980s. Equally, the 'liberal collectivist' view is generally representative of what has been described as the 'consensus' view of the post-war welfare state espoused by both Labour and Conservative governments in Britain up until the early 1970s. The different theorisations of the welfare role of the state are individually outlined in the following sub-sections.

THE REALITIES OF THE 'LIBERAL COLLECTIVIST' WELFARE STATE

In Britain, the post-war welfare state was built upon a politically liberal consensus (more or less upheld by both the major political parties up until the mid-1970s) that the role of the modern state should be directed towards mitigating the worst 'excesses' (or 'externalities' as they are sometime termed) of the market economy and providing some degree of security and equity for the citizens of a nation. This view was based on two main assumptions. First, that the state had the capacity and responsibility to intervene in the economy to ensure and maintain economic growth, and to maintain full employment in an open, yet regulated, market economy. Second, that only the state had both the resources to provide centralised and planned health and social services, free at the point of use, which would ensure the maintenance of the health and security of all its citizens.

The development of this post-war British welfare state was strongly associated with a concept of citizenship (addressed for the first time in British political history) that incorporated the principle of universal 'social rights' to be guaranteed by the rule of law. These 'social rights', in addition to pre-existing civil and political rights, were to serve as protection from the negative consequences of the market economy. This perspective had its roots in a tradition of political liberalism that was described

Table 2.1 Five key political-ideological conceptualisations of the role of the state in health and welfare provision

Socio-political theoretical explanation	The wider role of the state	Prescriptive health and welfare role of state	Implicit ideological and political values	Assessment of the balance between economic and social policies	Explanation of the cause of social and health problems
Liberal Collectivist *A perspective associated with the post-war political mainstream in the UK and EU countries*	As a neutral instrument	Guarantor of collective universal 'social rights' within an open market economy	Pragmatism; individual freedom within an efficient but fair capitalist economic system	Social policy used to redress inequities of market	Individual failure, combined with 'dysfunctions' of the economy
Neo-liberalism *A perspective associated with the political 'right' in the UK*	As an institution which perpetuates its own self-interests and which distorts the mechanisms of the free market	As minimal as possible, providing at best 'safety-net' provision and maintaining economic infrastructure	Libertarian; freedom of the market; 'free choice'	The market is distorted by state health and welfare interventions	Individual failure and inadequacy
Foucauldian *An influential academic perspective*	As having a regulatory and surveillance role	None	A critical analytical approach with no overt social and political values	An indeterminate notion of health leads to a rejection of the neo-liberal notion of health as a duty of citizenship	No government can ever provide the conditions under which all citizens have potentially equal chances for health
Political-economy *A perspective traditionally associated with the political 'left' in the UK*	The 'relatively autonomous' state seen as serving to maintain social cohesion and the long-term conditions for capital accumulation	Maximum intervention in the economy to reduce exploitation and reduce inequalities	Social equality; social harmony and justice; seeks to end or severely capitalist exploitation	Social policy means intervention in the market to ensure economic decisions take account of social responsibilities	Dysfunctions of capitalist economic system, plus maladministration of welfare state
Feminist *A perspective often missing from mainstream analysis and political debate*	Perpetuates patriarchal domination	Promote 'women-friendly' policies	End the male oppression of women in society	Some divergence on this question, reflecting different forms of feminism	For women – because they are denied the opportunity to participate equally in society

by T.H. Marshall (1950) as 'welfare capitalism', a form of governance that was seen to be able to deliver both national economic growth and social protection for its citizens.

The form of the state that characteristically emerged in this post-war period in Britain is often also referred to as the 'Keynesian Welfare State', named after the influential economist John Maynard Keynes, who, together with William Beveridge, were the leading architects of the British welfare state. It was Keynes who championed the need for the state to take on a much greater role in economic demand management to avoid a re-occurrence of the economic depression of the 1930s, which finally ended the myth of the market as being a self-regulating mechanism. The door was opened for a much more proactive role for state in providing health and welfare services to offset the dysfunctions of the market following the post-war election of the Labour government in 1945. Jessop (2000) has described the emergence of this new form of collectivist state welfare role as the 'Keynesian welfare national state' (KWNS). It being distinctively *Keynesian* in its focus on achieving full employment in a closed (as against global) economy by means of demand-side management. The *welfare* orientation is reflected in the linking of economic and social policies to a set of welfare rights associated with national citizenship. Finally it is *national* in that the Keynesian welfare policies are linked to a national territorial state (Jessop, 2000a: 173). However, with the downturn in the Western national economies in the early 1970s, all sorts of difficulties began to be experienced by the British welfare state. In response an alternative vision of the role of the state emerged from the political right, which is generally described as neo-liberalism and is described below.

NEO-LIBERALISM AND THE ROLE OF THE MARKET IN HEALTHCARE

Neo-liberalism as a political perspective became influential both in the USA and Britain in the mid-1970s, and whilst throughout the 1980s these ideas made little headway in France, Germany and the Nordic countries, by the end of the 1990s this perspective had become very influential within the EU. Neo-liberalism contends that countries with welfare states must inevitably experience economic crises because the monopoly provision of health and welfare services by the state leads directly to economic inefficiency. The tax burden of financing universal health and welfare services and benefits are seen to impact over time on the profitability of capital, as well as leading to social disincentives to individuals to take on greater personal responsibility. The solution was to reduce state welfare programmes to an absolute minimum, providing a safety-net of benefits only. This, neo-liberals argued, enabled tax reductions which could then be spent on personal consumption and re-investment in the market.

In Britain, this perspective was adopted ideologically (if not pragmatically) by the Conservative Party in the mid-1970s with the election of Margaret Thatcher as Party leader. Many claims have been made for the impact of the neo-liberal policies espoused by the Conservative government during its period of government between 1979 and 1997 in restructuring the health and welfare role of the state. Flinders (2006) has argued that, whilst there was not a reduction in the power of the state during this period, its health and welfare role was transformed; '(T)here has been a change in governing frameworks from hierarchical bureaucracies to complex networks and markets: a shift from govern*ment* to govern*ance* in which the extent of delegated responsibilities and the role of private contractors has increased' (Flinders, 2006: 224 – italics in original). Many of these neo-liberal ideas concerning the facilitating of 'public choices' by means of a widening of private sector involvement in service provision in order to stimulate greater efficiency and responsiveness to needs have been incorporated into the reforms of public services instigated by the New Labour government since coming to power in 1997 (discussed in detail in Chapter 9).

FOUCAULDIAN CONCEPTUALISATIONS OF THE REGULATORY ROLE OF THE STATE AS HEALTH PROVIDER

Over the past twenty-five years, the work of Michel Foucault has become very influential in the spheres of social, political and cultural analysis. Foucault developed the concept of 'governmentality' (or the 'art of government') in order to analyse the 'regulatory' (or interventionist) role of the state. This approach focuses attention on the ways in which power is present at all levels of society, serving to regulate the activities of the population (Foucault's conception of power, knowledge and discipline was described in Chapter 1). Foucault likened governmentality '… to a form of surveillance, of control which is as watchful as that of the head of a family over his household and his goods' (Foucault, 1979b: 10). As a conceptual tool, governmentality is primarily concerned with practices rather than institutions, with 'statecraft' or the 'space of government' rather than the formal workings of state institutions.

Therefore, for Foucault it is not possible to talk about a specific set of state policies directed at 'health', rather his work focuses upon the ways in which the health and behaviour of the population has increasingly become 'self-regulated'. Under neo-liberal state regimes in particular, where the market plays a much more important role in health provision, it becomes incumbent upon an individual member of the population to; '... enter into his or her own self-governance through processes of endless self-examination, self-care and self-improvement' (Petersen, 1997: 194). The direct role of government is limited to; '... constructing goals and targets in order to achieve strategically limited objectives ... (i)n response to the indeterminacy of health policy, neo-liberalism constructs the possibility of its strictly de-limited determination' (Osborne, 1997: 185). A good example of this approach would be the Conservative government's public health policy, *The Health of the Nation* policy (1992), which set out five strictly limited target areas for public health at the same time as specifying a whole range of personal and parental responsibilities. A similar set of targets was put forward in New Labour's own public health policy *Our Healthier Nation* (1998). As Petersen goes on to argue, the goals of this form of public health promotion strategy; '(h)ave, in effect, served the objective of privatising health by distributing responsibility for managing risk throughout the social body while at the same time creating new possibilities for intervention into private lives'(1997: 194).

THE POLITICAL-ECONOMIC CRITIQUE

This perspective, which is strongly influenced by a Marxist reading of class relations, has a very different reading of the historical development of state health and welfare policy. It recognises the welfare state as a particular historical form of the modern capitalist state, which has emerged in order to legitimate and thus reproduce existing capitalist social relations. In this regard, the universal provision of medical care for the population is seen as performing a very significant ideological function. As Lesley Doyal has argued, '(I)t is precisely because health, and therefore medical care, are so vital to every individual that the provision of medical care often comes to represent the benevolent face of an otherwise unequal and divided society' (1976: 43). However, this interventionist role of the state also has had negative consequences for the (capitalist) economy in terms of profitability. This paradoxical situation has been described in the following terms; '... while capitalism cannot coexist *with*, neither can it exist *without*, the welfare state' (Offe, 1984: 153 – emphasis in original).

The key themes of the political economy critique, found in the work of O'Connor (1973) and Gough (1979), is that state welfarism serves to build consent for capitalism through the process of dividing the population into discrete groups of 'clients', each with its own specific 'needs'. The state then offers welfare 'solutions' to these 'individual problems' via a plethora of state institutions and agencies. This has the effect of individualising what are actually widespread social and health problems associated with living in a capitalist society. Thus a common experience of poverty can be stood on its head through the construction of separate client groups, such as 'single parent families', the isolated elderly, people with a depressive illness, 'under-achieving children' and so on. A further critique is that the liberal collectivist welfare state has failed to meet the needs of all it its citizens equally despite the rhetoric. This is because the state in post-war Britain never intervened to tightly regulate the working of the market, so that pre-existing differentials in economic power between social groups were never addressed, the consequence of which was a widening health and income gap between social classes in Britain which continues up until the present day.

Some twenty-five years on, those theorists who continue to draw on this critique would recognise that the role of the welfare state has changed as the form of the national state has changed to match the needs of the national economy now operating within a globalised economic system. Jessop (1999) identifies a shift towards what he terms the 'international-isation of policy regimes'. That is, while the state provision of healthcare and welfare services for its citizens have not experienced the wholesale process of privatisation predicted by many commentators, this role is seen to have become increasingly subordinated to the national goal of promoting or 'regulating' greater economic innovation and 'international competitiveness' in the globalised economy. This analysis points to a new set of economic and social functions (not less) for the national state, and thus retains the political-economic critique focus on the importance of the accumulation requirements of the capitalist system in shaping the role of the national state.

FEMINIST CRITIQUE

Feminist critiques (acknowledging that there is no single form of feminism) of the health and welfare role of the state are largely predicated on the assumption that state welfarism serves to reproduce patriarchal domination within society, and so promote, albeit indirectly, women's oppression. Male domination of the 'public sphere' is seen as a form of determinism in policy-making. It sets the policy issue agenda, and excludes issues to do with the home and relationships (the 'private sphere') which are not regarded as legitimate areas for public discussion, for example child-rearing practices, domestic labour, and the predominant role of women as carers.

However, this view has been criticised as an overly radical form of Anglo-American feminism. It has been argued that the experience of women in the Nordic countries is very different as a consequence of the extensive system of 'women-friendly' policies adopted within the welfare states which arose as a direct consequence of social-democratic political principles of citizenship within these countries (Kantola, 2006). Hernes expresses this view as follows, 'In no other part of the world has the state been used so consistently by all groups, including women and their organisations, to solve collectively felt problems' (Hernes, 1988: 208). These Nordic welfare states are described as being 'women-friendly' because they assumed a dual-breadwinner model where both men and women were wage-workers (the premise that women's participation in the labour market was the key to gender equality), as against the single male 'family wage' model of liberal collectivist welfarism found in Britain. However, even here in the Nordic countries, as Hernes (1988) goes on to argue, women were essentially the object of policies executed by a male-dominated establishment, reinforcing a public dependency on the state.

ACTIVITY – THE ROLE OF THE STATE IN HEALTHCARE PROVISION IN CONTEMPORARY BRITAIN

Drawing upon the information provided in Table 2.1 (page 30) and upon your own additional reading (suggested list on page 37), what categories best fit the role of the state in healthcare provision as it is currently constituted?

Statement about the role of the state	Agree or disagree that this statement describes the current role of the state in healthcare provision within the UK, giving reasons
Guarantor of collective universal 'social rights' within an open market economy.	
As an institution which perpetuates its own self-interests and which distorts the mechanisms of the free market	
No government can ever provide the conditions under which all citizens have potentially equal chances for health.	
Maximum intervention in the economy to reduce exploitation and reduce inequalities.	
Perpetuates patriarchal domination.	
The 'relatively-autonomous' state seen as • serving to maintain social cohesion and the • long-term conditions for capital accumulation.	

CONCLUSIONS

The one general conclusion that can be drawn from the discussion of the five positions set out in the previous section, is that the welfare state within

Britain and other EU countries has undergone a significant restructuring over the past twenty years, and that this is an ongoing process. Whether this restructuring ultimately constitutes a significant shift in their founding liberal collectivist principles is something that is rather more difficult to agree upon. Neo-liberals and Foucauldians would both broadly agree that there has been a shift towards greater individual responsibility for personal health and welfare, although they disagree about whether this is something which has occurred because of a democratic impulse or a systemic process. Others such as the traditional liberal collectivists would argue that these moves towards citizens taking greater personal responsibility have been overstated. Whilst there is now a greater role for the market in health and welfare provision, this has occurred without challenging the set of political principles which guarantee the collective provision of health and welfare rights.

Analysts from the tradition of political economy would generally concur with the argument that there has been an erosion of the implicit contract between state and citizen, such that the latter has lost a trust in the ability of the welfare state to deliver universal services. Yet this is perceived to be less a mistrust of the welfare state *per se* (as neo-liberals would assert), than a disappointment with the perceived failure of state health and welfare provision to keep up with the public expectations. All major surveys of public opinion in Britain continue to find that the public hold the welfare state, and the NHS in particular, in high esteem.

SUMMARY

The aim of this chapter has been to explore the theoretically contested nature of the state and state power, and draw upon these conceptualisations in order to contextualise the development of the post-war welfare state. As can be ascertained from the outline of the key positions there is little common ground concerning the nature of state power, these differences are reflected in the five positions selected for detailed analysis set out in the second section of the chapter. There has been an attempt to delineate these contested theoretical positions through the use of two matrices. Figure 2.1 differentiates between the main state theories using the four dimensions of structure verses social agency, and 'state-made societies' as against 'society-made states', whilst Table 2.1 is concerned to map five major political-ideological theorisations of the role of the state in health and welfare provision in terms of a number of descriptive criteria. Both these representations are subject to challenge, but the aim has been to draw attention to the reasons why state and welfare theory is such a contested domain within the social and political sciences. It follows that an understanding of the theoretical assumptions underpinning the activities of the state is of central importance when engaging with the detailed discussion of health policy that appears throughout this text.

FURTHER READING

Hay, C., Lister, M. and Marsh, D. (eds) (2006) *The State: Theories and Issues.* Basingstoke: Palgrave Macmillan.

Pierson, C. (1996) *The Modern State.* London: Routledge.

Schumpeter, J. A. (1976) *Capitalism, Socialism and Democracy.* Harper and Row, New York.

Sharma, A. and Gupta, A. (eds) (2006) *The Anthropology of the State.* Oxford: Blackwell.

3   THE POLICY-MAKING PROCESS

CHAPTER CONTENTS

- Introduction
- Decision-making in bureaucratic organisations
- Ideal-type models of public policy decision-making
- Who sets the policy agenda?
- The implementation of policy
- A case study of policy implementation: Developing a patient-centred approach in General Practice
- Summary

INTRODUCTION

As has been discussed in the previous chapter, policy-making is fundamentally a political process involving the exercise of power. Therefore, any analysis of the health care policy process should assess not only the substance of a specific policy, but also the organisational processes and decision-making structures that are involved in initiating and implementing that policy. In turn, an assessment of the organisational *form* of the healthcare system, that is its hierarchical and regulatory structures, its division of labour, information processing systems and more, is also an essential prerequisite for health policy analysis.

Max Weber's classic model of an 'ideal-type' rational bureaucracy is a theoretical construction that has profoundly influenced and informed the understanding of organisational processes for over seventy years. This chapter outlines the main characteristics of this model and then moves on to develop a description of more recent (post-Weberian) ideal-type models of the public policy-making process. The intended function of these models is not only to explain, understand and interpret government policy-making, but also to prescribe the best way to decide between choices of political action. The final sections of the chapter examines the 'who' of the policy-making process, the key policy actors, identified as politicians and their political parties, pressure groups, and not least the state bureaucracy and policy networks. These all have to a greater or lesser extent the capacity or power to influence the policy decision-making process. This discussion moves onto an assessment of the 'how' of policy-making, the implementation process. It explores, through the use of a case study, why it is that the overarching objectives of policy-makers are not always delivered in practice.

DECISION-MAKING IN BUREAUCRATIC ORGANISATIONS

Historically, bureaucracies have been conceptualised both as rational and objective structures designed to efficiently achieve the goals of an organisation, or alternatively as self-serving Kafkesque labyrinthine institutions. Bureaucracies, unlike other social structures such as the family, communities, social networks of friends and peers, exist primarily to attain specific goals. In modern times, large bureaucratic organisations have arguably become the dominant social institutions within society; the most developed of which is the modern state apparatus.

The term 'bureaucracy' is often used in a pejorative sense to describe the ways in which complex organisational structures represent a rejection of an essential humanity in pursuit of a rationalist and technical solution to the demands of modern societies. This conception derives from the work of Max Weber, whose work on bureaucracy is now universally recognised as breaking the theoretical ground for the modern study of organisations. Underpinning Weber's work on bureaucracy was his general theory of social action, that all human action is determined by meanings and motives. In pre-modern societies, Weber recognised the social action of individuals and social groups as characterised by emotions, tradition and custom. But, in modern societies, such action is determined by rationality, which he defined as clear sets of goals and a systematic assessment of the means to achieve these goals. Weber identified the process of bureaucratisation as the prime example of the rationality of social action:

> Once fully established bureaucracy is among the structures which are hard to destroy. Bureaucracy is *the* means of transforming social action into rationally organized action. Therefore, as an instrument of rationally organized authority relations, bureaucracy was and is a power instrument of the first order for those who control the bureaucratic apparatus. Under otherwise equal conditions, rationally organized and directed action is superior to every kind of collective behaviour and also social action opposing it. Where administrations have been completely bureaucratized, the resulting system of domination is practically indestructible (Weber, 1978: 987 – cited in Eldridge, 1994: 94).

Writing in the early years of the twentieth century, Weber saw these rationalistic principles being applied in all the key arenas of a modern society, the market economy, technology, the law, and the state. Nevertheless, he was essentially pessimistic about what he saw as being an inexorable process in which the technically superior bureaucratic forms of organisation replaced all others. This was because the gradual encroachment of these types of organisations would effectively eliminate human difference and hence creativity; a loss of freedom to organisational and rational constraint. This essential pessimism was reflected in Weber's use of the term 'the iron cage' of bureaucracy; the 'discipline' of bureaucracy being seen to permeate all aspects of social and economic life.

For Weber, bureaucracy was a particular 'mode' or form of organisation. Historically, the defining characteristics of all organisations were that they consisted of a leader and administrative staff ordered into specific types of social relationship. This relationship was dependent upon the type of authority that was prevalent in any society at a particular time from which power (discussed in Chapter 1) was seen to derive. In modern societies, authority was seen to take the form of the rational-legal ideal type, encompassing the belief in the legality of patterns of normative rules, and the right of those elevated to authority under such rules to issue commands.

KEY CONCEPT – WEBER'S IDEAL-TYPE 'TENDENCIES' THAT CHARACTERISE BUREAUCRATIC ORGANISATIONS

a) A continuous organisation with a specified function, whose operations are governed by a system of abstract and formal rules, not by personal considerations;

b) Tasks are specific and distinct and carried out by formal categories of staff who specialise in certain specified tasks and not others;

c) The organisation of staff follows the principle of a hierarchy, with the rights and duties of officials at each level within the organisation specified;

(Continued)

(*Continued*)

d) Officials do not own any part of the organisation for which they work so that they cannot use their position for private gain; their official activities are quite separate from their private life;

e) Staff are appointed, not elected, on the basis of their specialist technical knowledge and expertise, and are promoted on the basis of merit;

f) Staff are paid salaries, with fixed terms of employment that specify what the qualities demanded for the job are. There is a clear career pathway;

g) Different positions within the hierarchy get differential pay and other benefits pertaining to their status within the organisation; a process of stratification;

h) Those with the power to issue commands are able to do so because the majority of the population are seen to accept the legal framework which supports this authority;

i) Obedience is not to the person who holds authority, but to the 'impersonal order' that has given this person this authority.

In any specific organisation, there may be more or less of any of these given tendencies. The typology of bureaucracy was conceptualised as an idealised representation that points to the types of processes that could be expected to be found if an organisation had bureaucratic tendencies. However, Weber's analysis of the spread of bureaucractic organisations should not be read as due solely to their efficiency; their development also represented for Weber the cultural constitution of the values of rationalisation as a structure of dominance in a modern society. Although contemporary organisational theory has largely moved away from Weber's instrumentalist account of bureaucratic organisational forms, his concerns with the cultural and institutional constitution of organisations as structures of dominant cultural values and ideology does represent an enduring legacy. Clegg's (1994) reworking of Weber's contribution in which he conceives bureaucratic rationality as primarily a set of discursive managerial practices, points to a key theme in the history of the NHS, the ongoing power conflict that has arisen between the individualised clinical discourse of healthcare professionals and the focus of healthcare management on the performance and efficiency of that organisation.

IDEAL-TYPE MODELS OF PUBLIC POLICY DECISION-MAKING

A competing range of what might best be described as post-Weberian ideal-type models of public policy emerged in the post-war period. Each of these models sees itself as reflecting a more realistic understanding of the functioning of public organisations than that attributed to the much maligned classic Weberian bureaucratic rationality model. The function of these models is to explain, understand, interpret and organise data concerning the making of decisions by government (Lane, 2000: 73). These models are also frequently normative ones, with their authors motivated by a desire to prescribe the best way to make policy decisions within public organisations such as the NHS (Hill, 1997: 98).

Simon's (1957) influential *rational decision-making model* is concerned with, '… the processes of decision as well as with the processes of action' (1957: 1). His model focused upon the common decision-making properties of organisations irrespective of their function. This approach emphasised the essential pragmatic rationality of organisations, in which decision-making was seen to be essentially a process that was concerned with selecting from a range of alternatives ranked in importance. The selection process was about choosing an option which maximised the attainment of the values of the organisation following a comprehensive analysis of the alternatives and their consequences. This required the prior setting-out of 'ends', and the identification of the 'means' of achieving these ends.

Whilst these common decision-making behaviours could be seen to reflect Weber's tendency to bureaucratisation, there was also an acknowledgement of the uncertainty associated with input flows in a general system, these were conceptualised by Simon as sources of change in the patterns of organisational behaviour (Clegg, 1994: 62). This was a conception of organisations as evolving 'organic' systems, which, whilst having formally rational internal structures, also had emergent properties from where dynamic change could arise. Simon (1957) also accepted that decision-making processes were not always rational because organisations could never be entirely homogeneous structures, and recognised that it was possible for the goals of individual decision-makers to differ from that of the organisation as a whole. Simon acknowledged the difficulties with the prior specification of ends and the identification of means to achieve these ends, recognising that the means cannot be easily separated from the values of the decision-makers themselves. On this basis, he conceded that only a limited or 'bounded rationality' was possible within public or state bureaucracies. This is because such public service organisations often lack the technical ability to ensure means achieve ends because the causal relationship between action (policy programmes) and desired outcomes is not a precise one, unlike in manufacturing organisations for example. This reflects the fact (missing in Simon's model) that the goals and values of state organisations are themselves policies and so are continually subject to dispute and change (Hill, 2004: 146).

Simon's rational decision-making model was challenged by authors such as Braybrooke and Lindblom (1963) who argued that in practice policy decisions were made incrementally. That is, organisational decision-making proceeds by limiting the number of policy alternatives to be considered to those only marginally different from existing policies. This *incrementalist model*, also known as 'muddling through', is said to be a consequence of the limited problem-solving capacities of many organisations. The limitations identified by Braybrooke and Lindblom (1963) include inadequate access to the appropriate information, failure to develop satisfactory evaluation and assessment methods, and the sheer multiplicity of variables within which the organisation operates.

Incrementalism was regarded by Braybrooke and Lindblom (1963) not only as an assessment of the policy-making process within organisations, but also an ideal-type prescriptive model of policy-making in pluralist societies. The authors asserted that serious mistakes could be avoided if only small changes are made in policy at any one time. They also went on to argue that the muddling-through model best suited the pluralistic policy process of bargaining and negotiation between different interest groups in the political system. Lindblom (1965) went on to address the question of how incrementalism operates in the public sector where there are many independent bureaucratic decision-makers. He argued that a process he termed 'mutual adjustment' occurs when local decision-makers seek to adapt to the decisions of others around them, whilst at the same time working to 'manipulate' the desired response from others within that organisation.

However, applied to public policy-making, the incrementalist model does have important deficiencies. The deductive power of the model is limited by the difficulties it faces when interpreting the concept of an 'increment', the size of changes that are made within policy. The model also assumes that decision-making processes are stable over time, and that future decisions are a linear function of the past. In practice, what are known as 'shift-points' or a fundamental rethinking about the course of policy development occur which defy such incrementalist equations (Lane, 2000: 76). Such shifts can occur when a new government with a radical political agenda comes into power, destabilising the policy process. An example of this process occurred in Britain with the election of Margaret Thatcher's Conservative Party in 1979 which immediately set about undermining post-war certainties with regard to the course of health and welfare policy.

Public choice theory has its origins in rational choice theory (discussed in relation to neo-liberal critique of the role of the modern state in Chapter 2), and asserts that the self-interest maximisation of policy actors acts as a key determinate of policy-making choices. An example of this process is found in the work of both Nordhaus (1975) and of Mueller (1979, 1989), where it is argued that incumbent governments will stimulate the economy before an election by increasing spending on programmes that appeal to the electorate (in order to get re-elected), and then deflate it after the election by raising taxes or reducing public deficits by some other means. Another critique of policy-making in state bureaucracies that draws on public choice theory can be found in the work of Tullock (1965, 1976) and Brittan (1977). Both writers argue that as a consequence of the need to respond to public demands, bureaucracies act to reinforce their own interests, thus growing in power and importance. However, this uncontrolled bureaucratic activity is ultimately deemed to result in enlarged state budgets and an expansion in the size of these bureaucratic organisations leading to the inefficient use of public resources.

Although public choice models do not lack political plausibility and have undoubtedly been very influential they often lack an empirical basis for their conclusions. The models also tend to over-emphasise the supply side in public policy-making. That is, they generally focus on what are seen to be excessive budget allocations for the supply of public goods and services, and not on the demands of the voters and the extent to which more socially deprived groups benefit through redistributive programmes transferring payments from high to low income groups (Lane, 2000: 90).

By the late 1970s, attempts to model governmental decision-making as a rational or linear incremental set of processes was increasingly being challenged by the emergence of what became known as the 'garbage can model' of policy decision-making (March and Olsen, 1976; Olsen, 1983). This model saw itself as a more realistic representation of constraints to rational policy-making within public organisations, which included ambiguous organisational values, uncertain knowledge about outcomes of decisions, and rules about decision-making which were largely politically symbolic. The model emphasised the apparent irrational and chaotic elements of organisational decision-making behaviour (and in doing so represented a complete rejection of the Weberian model of bureaucracy).

In conclusion, whilst there was once a consensus around a Weberian conception of politics and administration, no general theory of the policy decision-making process has emerged to replace it. Rather, as Lane has argued, there has been a proliferation of models broadly divided between rationalist and realist interpretations of the policy process, around which there is no consensus: 'The realist models of policy-making suggest no limit to the amount of complexity and number of variables to be taken into account (whilst) ... the simple models of rational policy making appear to be the only tools that give the policy analyst some direction where to look for explanations when policy-making deviates from model predictions' (Lane, 2000; 96).

WHO SETS THE POLICY AGENDA?

Having outlined a range of normative models of public policy decision-making, this section explores the role of the major players or 'policy actors' in setting the public policy agenda. These policy actors are identified as the political parties and politicians who set out policy programmes when standing for election to government; interest groups of all types from large and powerful corporate bodies through to single issue pressure groups run by volunteers to effect a particular policy change; and finally the state bureaucracy or, as it is more usually termed in Britain, the Civil Service.

A simplistic version of the pluralist model of democratic government would present policy-making as formally a transparent process. All the key policy actors would be seen as having a clearly specified role, with their contribution at each specified stage of the decision-making process being known. Within the British political system of government this policy process would, in theory, occur in the following way. The politicians, together with their advisors, transmute the political values and ideology of their political party into a series of policy proposals which are set out in an election manifesto. The political programmes of each political party contesting a general election are put to the electorate, and a government is formed by the Party whose programme is supported by the majority of the voting general public. Once in power, the new Party of government sets out its legislative programme (which in principle should match its election commitments), then a process of formal consultation follows during which pressure groups can lobby for their views to be incorporated. The final detailed proposals are then drawn up by senior civil servants and set out in a published 'White Paper', a final parliamentary debate then occurs followed by a vote in the House of Commons and the subsequent passing of legislation (an Act of Parliament). The new regulations are then enforced through guidance and formal instructions to State officials (senior civil servants). However, this simple constitutional model raises more questions than it answers. Issues of power are largely absent, and the rationality of the bureaucracy and its contribution to drawing up legislation is accepted at face value.

This analysis of the role of the three major groups of policy actors in setting policy agendas begins first with an examination of the role of political parties and politicians. As we have seen, the public choice model highlights the ways in which the role of politicians in setting the policy-making agenda may diverge substantially from the classic pluralistic model. The priority of politicians is to agree upon a party political programme that will get them elected to government, rather than one that is necessarily in accordance with the ideological values of their political party. Thus, policy issues which outwardly benefit the individual interests of the majority of the electorate are promoted, but at the cost of a concern with the long-term fiscal probity. A different perspective of the role of political parties in the policy process would be one that emphasised the continuing importance of political ideology in the setting of the policy agenda (see 'Ideology' as a *Key concept* in Chapter 2). As Hill (1997: 114) has noted, where a clear ideological difference exists and is contested between political parties competing for political office, the agenda-setting role of parties will be very evident in the early stages of policy-making. However, beyond this stage other policy actors become involved in the mediation or translation of these policy ideas into a firm set of proposals.

Interest groups are often able to play a decisive role in shifting the policy agenda in order to meet the specific interests or ideological values that they represent. Even small single issue pressure groups with limited resources can make an impact, particularly when they cluster together with other groups to form 'issue networks'. Within classic pluralist theory, as we have seen in the discussion of Dahl's work in Chapter 2, pressure groups are lauded as having a legitimate role in the democratic process in representing the diversity of interests that exist in modern societies. However, in contradistinction to classic pluralist theory, the political and economic interests of powerful elite groups within a society do not need to work through the political process in the way that single issue pressure groups are required to do. Powerful corporate interest groups are frequently able to directly negotiate with politicians and state officials outside the formal consultative machinery of government. It has been reported that in the USA more than 35,000 professional lobbyists in support of private commercial interests now spend at least $5bn every year trying to influence the votes of members of the US Congress ('Cracks in an evil edifice', Leader, *The Guardian*, 9th January 2006). In the British political system such forms of lobbying may not be quite as developed, but it does point to the importance of policy-making processes which are located outside any formal process of representative democracy.

The third key policy actor is the state bureaucracy itself. The key role of senior civil servants in the policy process has been discussed above in relation to models of bureaucratic organisation. And as Weber himself recognised, the inherent danger associated with such organisations is that the bureaucrats themselves often seek to become their own masters. Whilst the role of senior civil servants is formally that of providing the expertise for detailed problem-solving, often this role can become more than one of adjusting policy at the pre-implementation stage; civil servants can and do make substantive 'improvements' in a policy. As we have seen in the discussion of the key concept of power (see Chapter 1), Steven Lukes (1974: 2005) identified the second 'face of power' as being the ability to prevent particular issues being placed on the policy agenda or to prevent decisions being taken. State bureaucracies have the capacity to manipulate policy inputs in this way in order to maintain control over the policy process. In practice it is not possible to confine civil servants to a purely non-political administrative role because there is no clear distinction between ends and means in public policy-making such that it becomes impossible to separate politics from administration.

Another key issue surrounding the policy actor role of state bureaucracies concerns their political and ideological neutrality. In the past, as we have seen in the discussion of C. Wright Mills (1956) work on social elites, the social ties between the top state bureaucrats, business leaders and establishment figures were identified as particularly problematic for the democratic representational process. Today the issue tends not to be so much about the emasculation of radical political agendas by a politicised bureaucracy, as a concern with the 'policy communities' that involve the interaction between top personnel within the civil service and those from private corporations. This is particularly the case when there is ever greater market involvement in the provision of public goods and services. These issues surrounding the role of the key policy actors and the stage at which they become involved in the policy process leads us on to the discussion of the policy implementation process.

THE IMPLEMENTATION OF POLICY

The concept of implementation can be conceived as being essentially an ambiguous one, in that implementation refers both to the bringing about of an outcome, as well as to this outcome being consistent with the original intentions of the policy-makers. A policy that is executed need not necessarily result in the accomplishment of the policy objectives (Lane, 2000: 98). The policy literature once traditionally blurred the distinction between the policy-making process and its implementation and all too readily assumed that once a policy has been decided upon it would automatically achieve its objectives. The gradual realisation (by the mid-1970s) that there was a distinct lack of correspondence between policy objectives and policy outcome resulting from an 'implementation deficit', led to the development of a variety of 'implementation models' to provide a link between the policy process and the execution of that policy. The range of implementation models that have subsequently been developed are usually demarcated according to whether they emphasise a top-down or bottom-up approach to explaining the implementation deficit problem.

Top-down models are in essence ideal-types which seek to provide guidelines for those at the top of the policy-making process in order to minimise implementation problems. Hood's (1976) model focuses attention on the relations of authority in an organisation, which he sees as the primary mechanism for successful implementation of policy. The model seeks to identify the limits to control inherent in complex public administrative systems so that they can be more effectively managed. Similarly, Sabatier and Maznanian's (1979) work advises that a policy decision must contain unambiguous policy directives and implementation structures, whilst those charged with implementation should possess 'substantial managerial and political skills' and are committed to the policy goals (1979: 484–485). Hogwood and Gunn (1984) in turn set out ten preconditions they perceived as necessary for the achievement of perfect implementation.

The problem with many of these top-down models is that they presume a 'one-shot' process that involves the implementation in its entirety of a clear-cut entity, 'the policy'. In practice, policies are highly complex phenomena which can involve purely symbolic (as well as practical) elements, many of which politicians may have no intention of actually implementing. In addition, the implementation of a policy is often marked by a series of negotiations and compromises with conflicting sets of interests, ongoing throughout the life of a policy (Hill, 2004: 180). Where policies have been enacted in line with the formal bureaucratic top-down rule structures of government, without negotiation or compromise, they have often faced huge implementation problems. One outstanding example of such a failed policy is the Poll Tax, introduced by the Conservative government in the late 1980s, which on its implementation faced a mass campaign of civil disobedience and was subsequently replaced with a more measured reform. In practice, as Hill (2004: 182) has also noted, it is difficult to determine where the formal policy-making process ends and implementation begins, and he cites the following reasons for this assertion:

- Because conflicts of interest cannot be resolved at the policy-making stage;

- Because key decisions can only be made when all the facts are available to policy implementers;
- Because certain groups of implementers (professional managers, for example) are better equipped to make key decisions;
- Because policy-makers can only make educated guesses about the actual impact of new policies;
- Because it is recognised that the day-to-day task of implementation inevitably involves negotiation and compromise with powerful groups affected by the policy;
- Because it is considered politically inexpedient for central government to intervene to resolve the local conflicts arising out the implementation of national policy.

The alternative to the top-down models of the implementation process are bottom-up models. These models claim much greater realism in their description of the complexities associated with the process of implementation, having no predetermined theoretical assumptions. Elmore's (1982) 'backward mapping' approach argued that attention should be focused not upon the bureaucratic hierarchies but upon the 'concrete behaviour' of those lower down the hierarchy charged with actually carrying out policy. This is because at 'street level', actors charged with the implementation of a policy are often faced with making choices between programmes that may conflict or interact with one another (see the case study outlined below).

The question of the discretion available to policy actors in the implementation process and how this is structured is a central feature of both implementation models. Bottom-up models emphasise the importance of the trust placed by the public on the policy implementers who require a degree of freedom in order to handle the uncertainties associated with implementing new policies. While top-down models probably over-emphasise the responsibility of politicians and senior bureaucratic officials to the public in ensuring that outcomes match policy objectives. The bottom-up model commends spontaneity, learning and adaptation as problem-solving techniques for effective policy implementation, while the top-down recommends greater control, planning and hierarchy (Lane, 2000: 110). This reinforces the pertinence of the point made at the beginning of this section concerning the ambiguity of implementation as both the end-stage of the policy process, as well as being a stand alone process. Policy programmes are not all of one type, some have clear single aims whilst others are more innovative and complex. In this sense then, neither of the two main implementation models is satisfactory, yet the search for a universal model is probably an illusionary one. The process of policy-making needs to contextualised at a number of levels, and not only in terms of possible deficits in relation to the original policy objectives.

A CASE STUDY OF POLICY IMPLEMENTATION: DEVELOPING A PATIENT-CENTRED APPROACH IN GENERAL PRACTICE

The promotion of the principles of patient-centred primary care by the Department of Health pre-dated the coming to power of the New Labour government; although it fully encouraged this development in-line with its widening patient choice agenda. The patient-centred care management approach seeks to promote the identification of the specific needs of the patient through a process of negotiation as being a clinical priority. The evidence is that this approach does improve patient adherence to their medication regime (Royal Pharmaceutical Society of Britain, 1997). The patient-centred approach to prescribing would assert that the effective risk management of a condition such as coronary heart disease is dependent not only upon clinicians systematically identifying and treating those at risk with appropriate medication, but that it also requires the direct involvement of the patient exercising some measure of personal control and choice over their treatment.

In 2000, the Department of Health published its Coronary Heart Disease (CHD) National Service Framework (NSFs as a central feature of New Labour's 'modernisation' of the NHS policy are discussed in detail in Chapter 8) which sets out 12 standards for the prevention, diagnosis and treatment of the disease (DoH, 2000c). Standard Number 3 of the NSF recommended that GPs identify and develop a register of diagnosed patients and those patients at high risk of developing CHD. Dietary and lifestyle advice (what the document terms 'modifiable risk factors') is to be offered to these patients, and their medication reviewed at least every 12 months. It was also recommended that statins be prescribed to anyone with CHD or having a 30 percent or greater ten-year risk of a 'cardiac event', in order to lower their blood cholesterol levels to less than 5 mmol/l or by 30 percent (which ever is greater). These recommendations acquired teeth when they were incorporated into the new Quality and Outcomes Framework (QOF) that identified clinical indicators and targets for a list of disease categories which Primary Care Organisations were now required to meet. The QOF framework formed the centrepiece of the General Medical Services contract agreed by GPs that came into operation in 2003. The relative performance of an individual Primary Care Practice in meeting each of these indicators now attracts points on a sliding scale that are then converted into payments for individual GPs. In relation to the management of patients with CHD, higher payments are received if the practice increases the percentage of its patients who have their total serum cholesterol regularly monitored, and whose last cholesterol reading was less than 5 mmol/l (DoH, 2004d).

The introduction of these incentivised CHD NSF guidelines (as well as those of other NSF's) have arguably served to nullify the widespread adoption of a patient-centred approach in General Practice. The possibilities for patient-centred care being overwhelmed by the requirements of the reform process that seeks to achieve a more cost-effective and performance-led healthcare system:

... (S)uch a conclusion should not be read as implying that the widespread introduction of systematic monitoring and statin therapy is of no therapeutic benefit to people living with coronary heart disease, indeed it is clear that it has prolonged the lives of many patients. Rather, the purpose is to draw attention to the potential consequences of GPs singularly following (financially incentivised) national risk management guidance (Crinson et al., 2007: 12).

So for example, the regular titrating of the dose or frequency of a statin or anti-hypertensive drug prescription can lead to a decrease in adherence to a medication regime over time .(Dowell and Hudson, 1997; Whitney, 1993). Another study of clinicians and lay people's attitudes towards taking medication for secondary preventative purposes also concluded that the CHD NSF represented an imposition of inflexible national guidelines that served to marginalise patient's own treatment preferences (Lewis, Robinson and Wilkinson, 2003).

This case study illustrates the way which the practical process of policy implementation in a complex structure such as the NHS, whether intentional or not, can contradict and undermine previous policy goals. Whether this is an example of the Braybrooke and Lindblom (1963) incrementalist model is open to question, but the failure to take into account the consequences of introducing incentivised performance payments for the doctor-patient relationship does point to this being an example of 'muddling through'.

ACTIVITY

This exercise is designed to encourage you to reflect upon the policy decision-making discussion set out in this chapter, and also as preparation for the next chapter on the structure of healthcare in Britain. Identify a recent policy development in the NHS that has run into difficulties between the policy formulation and implementation stages; for example the development of community-based 'polyclinics' or the widening patient choice agenda. Then briefly describe the factors that you think have played a part in this process.

SUMMARY

This chapter has examined a range of policy-making ideal-typologies, some of which are normative in intent. Such ideal- typologies do serve an important function in drawing attention to common characteristics of the phenomena being studied (in this case, public policy-making processes) which enable comparative analyses of different forms of healthcare system. However, it is important to bear in mind that the uncritical application of ideal-typologies will often ignore the specific set of social and cultural contexts as well as political restraints which face public policy decision-makers. Here, Michael Hill (2004) makes the point that it is only during the process of implementation that a particular policy will actually become 'concretized', reflecting the political realities present at the time; this again points to the importance of studying policy context in addition to identifying common characteristics of the process.

The chapter has also attempted to reflect the previous discussion of power (see Chapter 1) in its assessment of the construction and implementation of public policy. So for example, Lukes' third dimension of power which draws attention to the way in which power can be exercised through the manipulation and shaping of the wants, needs and values present within a society, offers an important reminder that we should retain a critical assessment of the overarching objectives of government in the development of particular policies. This point was also addressed by Lindblom (1977) who, although an early initiator of the incrementalist model, later revised his essentially pluralistic view of the policy process and acknowledged that certain values and beliefs emanating from dominant or powerful groups can attain homogeneity or 'taken-for-granted' status within a society shaping the policy process. These are important considerations that should be borne in mind when we examine the development of the structure of the healthcare system in the next section of the book.

FURTHER READING

Cabinet Office Strategic Policy Making Team (1999) *Professional Policy Making for the Twenty-First Century*. Available at: www.policyhub.gov.uk/docs/profpolicymaking.pdf

Hill, M. (2004) *The Public Policy Process.* (4th Edn). Harlow: Pearson Longman.

Lane, J. E. (2000) *The Public Sector: Concepts, Models and Approaches* (3rd Edn). London: Sage.

PART TWO

THE HEALTHCARE SYSTEM

4 THE STRUCTURE OF HEALTHCARE IN THE UK: CONTINUITY AND CHANGE

INTRODUCTION

The founding of the NHS sixty years ago created a state funded system of universal healthcare, replacing the disorganised mixture of charity, local government, and private market provision which had existed before the Second World War. For nearly thirty years there was a broad political consensus that a central command and control system funded from direct taxation was the best means of delivering healthcare provision in Britain. However, in the thirty years since the mid-1970s, the relationship between the state and its citizens in relation to healthcare provision has been subject to ongoing political deliberation.

While the role of the private market in healthcare provision (known euphemistically as the 'independent sector') has remained a relatively limited one, the private sector and the economic principles of the market have always played a role in the provision of healthcare within the UK. This role expanded following the 'internal market' reforms of the Conservative government in 1990, and since its coming to power in 1997, The New Labour government has continued to extend the scale of this purchaser–provider division, encouraging the private sector and private finance to expand their role in the NHS.

This chapter begins by historically contextualising the development of the role of the state in healthcare provision in Britain, and goes on to trace the organisational transitions that have occurred since the foundation of the NHS in 1948. One section of the chapter is given over to an examination of the structure of NHS as it exists in Scotland, Wales and Northern Ireland. From its inception in 1948, there have been important differences in the organisational structures of the NHS have existed between these countries. These differences have widened significantly following the process of devolution of power from Westminster to the National Assemblies in Wales and Northern Ireland, and to the Scottish Parliament that occurred at the end of the 1990s.

THE HISTORICAL BACKGROUND TO THE DEVELOPMENT OF THE NHS

State involvement in the regulation and control of all the activities, resources and institutions of the nation has increased dramatically over the past century in Britain. In accounting for the development of this interventionist role, particularly in ensuring the provision of health and welfare services for all its citizens, the literature would point to the historical requirement for the state to overcome or limit the consequences ('externalities') of the drive for accumulation and competition that characterises the capitalist market in modern societies. The economic system is seen to require the intervention of what has been termed a 'collective actor' in order to provide the extensive infrastructure (transport, energy, availability of a skilled and healthy workforce, etc.) it needs in order to facilitate the production and distribution of commodities. Additionally, in order for the capitalist economic system to maintain its legitimacy amongst the population and ensure social stability, it also needs a collective 'safety net' (a system of social security or 'social protection') for those who are unable to earn an independent living, such as the long-term sick, those with physical or learning disabilities, and those who give up work to look after dependants. These functional requirements of the economic system it is argued eventually led onto the development of the 'welfare state.' This form of the state emerged in virtually all modern industrialised nations (with the notable exception of the USA) during the second half of the twentieth century.

Whilst acknowledging the centrality of this political-economic explanation of the emergence of the 'welfare state role', there are also national contextual factors that account for the particular form that state health and welfare provision takes in different countries. The direct involvement of the post-war state in Britain in health and social care provision arose because the fragmentary mix of 'voluntary' (or charity) hospitals, local government, and private market provision failed to comprehensively meet the healthcare needs of all members of the population. It is generally accepted that the inadequacy of healthcare provision was so apparent that a broad political consensus for radical change had been building even before the outbreak of the Second World War. Nevertheless, the requirements of the War gave this process a dramatic push forward.

The pre-war patchwork of services reflected the development of quite distinct forms of healthcare provision which had emerged historically in order to meet the needs of quite separate social groups. The private hospital sector (the 'voluntary hospitals' as they were known) had been established for well over a century, and included many of the more famous London hospitals such as Guy's, St Thomas's, the Middlesex, and St George's. Although these hospitals were formally charitable institutions, admission was selective and the poor were often denied access. By the 1930s these hospitals were experiencing severe financial problems. The major London hospitals derived only a third of their income from voluntary donations, and this was despite the increasing number of what were known as 'flag days' when medical staff went out to openly solicit money from the public. Other charitable organisations provided various community health services, particularly those that focused on the welfare of children and mothers.

The pre-war provision of health services for those who could not afford private treatment was organised through the local government authorities. These public bodies had inherited a hospital service which grew out of the nineteenth century system of relief for the poor and the destitute. In this 'Poor Law' system, harsh conditions were imposed upon all those seeking relief (starkly portrayed in many of the books of Charles Dickens). This followed from the principle of 'less eligibility' established by Chadwick in 1834 which required that any relief received must be worked for (within 'workhouses') and be at a level below the living standard of those in employment. However, this nineteenth century system did lead onto the foundation of Poor Law infirmaries, rudimentary hospitals for the 'sick poor', which were the first publicly funded form of healthcare provision.

The First World War exposed the poor physical condition of the working classes in Britain: only one in three conscripts for the armed forces was deemed fit enough to serve. This revelation led to the establishment of the first Ministry of Health in 1919 which was charged with integrating the different agencies providing health services to the public and reducing their deficiencies, particularly in child and maternity care. However, under the auspices of this new Ministry, the aforesaid public hospital service developed in only a piecemeal way in the inter-war period. Although local authorities were empowered in 1929 to take over the Poor Law infirmaries, few authorities outside of London seized this opportunity to create municipal hospitals. Between 1921 and 1938, the public provision of hospital beds increased by only 4000 to 176,000, with the voluntary hospitals providing a further 87,000 (Fraser, 1973: 186).

Alongside these developments in provision, a system of National Health Insurance based on individual contributions had been created in 1911, administered by local insurance committees ('Panels'). This scheme provided access to free GP services, sickness benefits and medications. However, the scheme only covered only those in employment, dependents were excluded from its benefits. With the mass unemployment of the 1930s, many workers lost their rights to these healthcare benefits.

THE NATIONAL HEALTH SERVICE 1948–1989

The sacrifices made by the population as a whole during the Second World War, particularly during the heavy bombing of the major cities in Britain, dramatically moved forward the political question of the government giving a commitment to playing a much more direct role in health service provision. At the very beginning of hostilities, the national government had set up the Emergency Hospital Service (EHS) to coordinate the work of all hospitals, private and local government, in anticipation of mass civilian causalities. Then, in 1941, the Ministry of Health announced that the economist William Beveridge had been commissioned to produce a report examining the ways in which a comprehensive social security and healthcare system could be created after the war. The Beveridge Report was published in 1942 and proposed the creation of a national welfare state which would provide a minimum standard of living 'below which no one should be allowed to fall', and in addition a National Health service providing medical treatment for 'all citizens'. The ensuing debate that followed the publication of the Report between the established interest groups in healthcare (hospital consultants and GPs, private insurance companies, the voluntary hospitals, as well as the local authorities) then became focused on just how these interests could or would be protected in a new comprehensive state health service.

Following the Labour Party's landslide victory in the 1945 general election at the end of the war, the ground was laid for the creation of a new form of welfare state on the lines proposed by Beveridge. The National Health Service (NHS) came into operation in July 1948, with the goal of providing a national comprehensive universal service, free at the point of delivery. The main funding mechanism for this new national service was to be through general taxation. However the system of National Insurance contributions established at the time only ever representing a fraction of the total cost of operating all the institutions of welfare including the NHS (see Chapter 5 for a detailed examination of funding). The local authority and private voluntary hospital services that existed pre-war were effectively nationalised and placed under central government control. One of the major stumbling blocks to the passing of the National Health Service Act of 1946, was the opposition of important sections of the medical profession. In order to facilitate a settlement, important concessions were made by the Labour government, GPs were able to retain their privileged position as independent contractors (and were not to become state employees), whilst hospital consultants were able to continue to retain their lucrative private practices whilst working within the new NHS. The opportunity afforded by the establishment of this new system of healthcare to challenge the principle of clinical autonomy (or 'clinical freedom' as the British Medical Association at the time liked to call it) was never taken up by the new Ministry of Health. Indeed, far from challenging the position of authority which the medical profession had established for themselves in the pre-war system of healthcare, new powers were ceded to them, particularly in relation to resource allocation. This was a position of power within the NHS that the medical profession retained for over half a century (see Chapter 7).

The new NHS had a 'tripartite' organisational structure (see Figure 4.1). This included, 'Executive Councils' which took over from the pre-war private insurance panels and were given the responsibility of managing the contracts of 'family practitioners' (the generic name for GPs, dentists, opticians and pharmacists). Local Authorities were given the responsibility for delivering the range of environmental and personal health services (maternity and child welfare clinics, vaccination, health visitors, health education, and the ambulance service), While 'Regional Hospital Boards' (RHBs) administered the nationalised hospital sector. This tripartite structure reflected the divisions in the provision of healthcare that largely remain to this day. That is, between *primary* (preventative, involving GPs and community nurses), *secondary* (acute medicine, located in the Hospital sector), and *tertiary* (care of chronically ill); with the secondary care sector receiving the vast bulk of the resources.

One of the major criticisms levelled (in hindsight) at this organisational structure was that the control over spending and resources was effectively devolved to the medical profession. This ultimately had important consequences for the equitable distribution of resources across the NHS, and impeded the development of a more cost-effective service. Although the new Minister of Health, Aneurin Bevan, had played a crucial role in sustaining the principles of a comprehensive healthcare system during the long gestation period before the final establishment of the NHS, largely through the force of his dominant personality and political convictions,

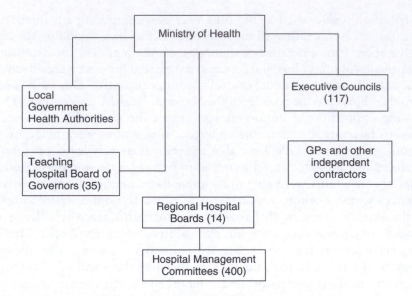

Figure 4.1 The 1948 organisational structure of the NHS

he did fail to ensure that an effective and powerful administrative structure was put in place to ensure that these principles were carried through (Lowe, 1993: 179).

Although the acute hospital or secondary care sector received the largest proportion of resources in the new NHS, it was argued at the time that twentieth-century medicine was being practised in nineteenth-century buildings. This was primarily a legacy of the under-funded, ill-equipped, and unevenly distributed pre-war provision of health services. It was not until the 1960s that the state was in a financial position to be able to provide the additional resources that were urgently needed in order to expand and update these hospitals. It was also not until the 1960s that any form of strategic planning for the GP primary care service was undertaken. The pre-war distribution of GPs had always been patchy, yet twenty years after the founding of the NHS, 33 million people were still considered to be living in 'undoctored' areas, particularly in the inner city areas (Ham, 1992: 20). Although GPs could not be forced to practice in any particular area of the country, financial inducements were introduced to try and overcome the imbalance in primary care provision together with the priority attached to the building of new 'health centres'.

The structure of the NHS was administratively (rather than politically) re-organised in 1974; this process had three main aims. Firstly, to integrate local health services under one Area Health Authority (AHA) previously administered by the RHBs, local government, and Hospital Boards of Governors. Secondly, to achieve better coordination between Health authorities and local authorities. Thirdly, to achieve more efficient management structures by introducing multi-disciplinary teamwork, consensus management, and to involve doctors in the day-to-day management of the service. Even as these changes came on-stream, criticisms of the organisational structure were beginning to build. In particular there were increasing delays in decision-making reflecting the poor relationships that existed between the many administrative tiers that existed in the restructured organisation. The opportunity to more closely integrate the various healthcare sectors was not seized, and the Executive Committees for GPs, dentists and opticians were excluded from the remit of the new AHAs, and remained separate under the new Family Practitioner Committees (FPCs) which replaced the Executive Committees. Although responsibility for the provision of community health services (district nursing and midwifery services within the community) was transferred to the NHS from local authorities, the latter retained control over environmental health and social care services. In effect, the tripartite division of health services continued following this re-organisation, a structure that effectively discouraged the integration of health and social care services between the NHS, local authorities and the FPCs.

In 1976 the Labour government was faced with a deterioration in public support following its failure to address the under-funding of the NHS. The perceived lack of commitment to NHS staff had led to serious industrial relations problems, not only around the issue of low pay, but also the introduction of private 'pay beds' into hospitals. The government in response established a Royal Commission on the NHS to look into the management of financial and manpower resources. The recommendations of the Merrison Commission (1979) were finally published shortly after the election of a new Conservative government headed by Margaret Thatcher in 1979. Whilst the final report endorsed the founding principles of the NHS, it condemned what it saw as the excessive bureaucracy of the organisation and argued that the performance of the organisation could be improved through greater efficiency. The Report also for the first time identified the existence of widening social and geographical inequalities in health, but recognised that this was a social problem that could not be addressed by the NHS in isolation. While the recommendations concerning inequalities in health were essentially ignored, the new Conservative government did produce its own response to the recommendations concerned with the organisational structure of the NHS. *Patients First* (DHSS, 1979b) recommended the abolition of the middle administrative tier of the Area Health authorities (which had only been in place for eight years). This tier was subsequently abolished in 1982, leaving Regional and District Health Authorities with the responsibility for the planning and implementation of policy.

Although the Conservative government was to go on to carry through a far more radical re-organisation of the NHS, this did not occur until a decade later. Initially the focus of the government in relation to the NHS was to build on the concerns of the Royal Commission about the need to address organisational performance and control over public spending. Following the recommendations of an inquiry team set up by the DHSS and headed by Sir Roy Griffiths, the managing director of Sainsbury's supermarket chain, a series of reforms of the managerial and decision-making structures within the organisation was proposed. This Griffiths Inquiry Report (DHSS, 1983) has been highly critical of the consensus form of management that had predominated in the organisation over the previous decade, arguing that this resulted in a blurring of the lines of responsibility and a failure to take tough decisions about resource spending. This 'consensus management' was favoured by doctors on account of the high degree of control over decision-making that they were able to exercise, and by nurses because it had elevated their status in the management structure (Webster, 2002: 173). The inquiry also identified a problem in the relationship that existed between the DHSS (the government Ministry responsible for strategic health planning) and the NHS (the organisation charged with delivering healthcare for the population). The report argued that there was too much top-down directing of the day-to-day management of the health service by Whitehall. The main recommendations of the Griffiths report were concerned with the replacing of consensus management with a system of general management applied to all levels of the NHS. However, as Webster has noted, although there was much talk about recruiting these new general managers from private industry, most management appointments subsequently went to senior administrators working with health authorities and hospitals (2002: 173).

REFORMING THE STRUCTURE OF THE NHS: 1990 AND BEYOND

Although the changes that had been instigated in local management decision-making structures had marked an important step in achieving greater efficiencies in the delivery of health services, they could not compensate for the years of resource under-funding within the NHS (which had a significantly lower level of expenditure on healthcare than other equivalent European countries). In the face of an increasing public dissatisfaction with the failure of the NHS to meet the growing demands upon the health service that derived not only from the demographic changes in society, but also rising expectations about the type of service the public should be receiving, the Conservative government instigated a major process of structural reform.

Throughout the 1980s, the Prime Minister, Margaret Thatcher, had not held back from reform in most sectors of the welfare state, but she had been reluctant to introduce a radical market-led reform of the NHS given the generally high levels of popular support it enjoyed. After nearly a decade in power, she could no longer avoid the political pressure to address the perceived malaise in the health service. In January 1988, the Prime Minister announced, via an interview on the BBC *Panorama* programme, that she was setting-up a high-level inquiry. This review was predicated on the assumption that the NHS continued to be an inflexible bureaucratic organisation unable to respond to change, reflecting the undiminished and unchallenged clinical decision-making power and autonomy of the hospital consultants and GPs. Despite the introduction of the 'general management' in the mid-1980s, the organisation was perceived to have failed to provide the incentives necessary for staff to achieve greater 'efficiency'; no sanctions had ever been applied to hospitals with above average costs. Nationally negotiated working conditions and pay for all grades of staff were also seen as a factor in restricting the flexibility of local managers to address local pressures and demands. The ethos of the health service was perceived by the Conservative government's review to be 'provider-dominated' with little concern for the needs of patients. The review concluded that there was insufficient public accountability for the costs and the quality of healthcare delivery. The outcome of this review was the *Working for Patients* White Paper (DoH, 1989a) published in January 1989.

Working for Patients, described by the Prime Minister Margaret Thatcher as 'the most far-reaching reform of the NHS in its forty year history' (cited in Webster, 2002: 190), proposed a series of radical changes to the structure of the NHS which became known as the 'internal market' reforms. These structural changes sought to bring about a separation of the purchasing of healthcare from its provision. Hospitals were encouraged to opt out of DHA control and become self-governing Trusts, and as such were allowed to compete as providers and win contracts from the purchasers, the local Health Authorities and the new 'fundholding' GP practices. The latter were those GP practices that took the 'opportunity' now available to them of being allocated a top slice of the local DHA budget in order to purchase a range of health services for their own patients. The reforms also introduced mandatory quality assurance systems, and restructured the NHS executive and regional health authorities (see Figure 4.2).

The criticism of the *Working for Patients* 'internal market' proposals made at the time was that the reform process had been rushed through too quickly, with little attention paid to the detailed development of the new set of contractual arrangements between DHAs, GP practices and Health Authorities. The reaction to the reforms from the health professions was vociferous, Klein describing it as the 'biggest explosion of political

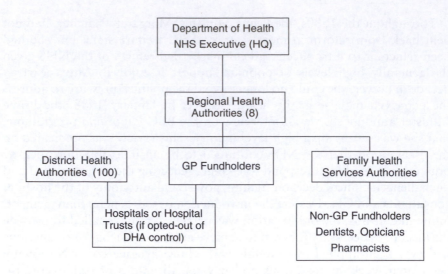

Figure 4.2 The 1989 organisational structure of the NHS

anger and professional fury in the history of the NHS' (Klein, 1995: 131, cited in Webster, 2002: 194). The British Medical Association (BMA) launched a campaign of opposition against the White Paper proposals, and were supported in this by other health service trade unions as well as the Opposition Labour Party. However, the Secretary of State for Health, Ken Clarke, refused to make any concessions and the BMA eventually called off their campaign in mid-1992. As the reforms were rolled out across the organisation, it became apparent to the BMA that, whilst the internal market reforms certainly challenged important principles of equity of access to health services, ultimately they were not fundamentally detrimental to the professional interests of their members. Nevertheless, at the grass roots level of general practice, many groups of doctors continued to resist the inducements being offered by the NHS Executive to become fundholding practices. By the time of the General Election in 1997, which brought an end to eighteen years of Conservative government rule, nearly half of all general practices remained non-fundholding.

The introduction of 'internal market' mechanisms into the structure of the NHS following the NHS and Community Care Act (1990), and the subsequent development of what was termed a 'two-tier health service' (fundholding practices finding it easier to refer their patients to specialist hospital services) appeared at the time to challenge the universalist principles of the NHS. However, the notion of an 'internal market' was essentially a hybrid construct imposed from above upon a healthcare system which continued to remain free at the point of use. This resulted in an organisational structure where, as Webster describes it:

> 'Internal' was clearly inconsistent with the aspiration to maximise the involvement of outside agencies and the private sector. The 'market' analogy was obviously imprecise, since the consumer was unable to exercise choice of services; health authorities or fundholders acted as their surrogates. It was not so much a matter of the patient dictating where the money went, but the patient following whatever channel the professionals dictated (Webster, 2002: 202)

Over time questions began to arise as to political commitment of the Conservative government in pursuing their ideological goal of encouraging private market penetration of the state healthcare system. Certainly these market principles barely penetrated the bureaucracy of the NHS and the day-to-day activities of healthcare professionals. As Rudolf Klein has argued:

> The notion driving these changes was that competition among providers to secure contracts either from the Health Authorities or from general practitioners who chose to be fund-holders would improve efficiency and responsiveness. For a variety of reasons, among them the reluctance of the government to give free rein to market forces, the reforms never functioned as intended (Klein, 2004: 937)

On being to returned to power in 1997 after eighteen years in opposition, New Labour began to set out its 'modernisation' programme for the NHS. The stated objective of the first White Paper on health service reform, *The New NHS: Modern, Dependable* (DoH, 1997a) introduced by the new government, was to gain more effective control and regulation over the use of healthcare resources so that the political goal of an 'efficient and equitable' health service could become achievable. The organisational structure of this 'modernised' NHS is set out in Figure 4.3. The modernisation programme also introduced new national regulatory instruments for the setting and monitoring of clinical standards and performance. These included the Commission for Health improvement (CHI), the National Institute of Clinical Excellence (NICE), as well as a public health strategy (*Our Healthier Nation*: DoH, 1998a) which sought for the first time to directly address social inequalities in health.

Probably the single most important structural reform initiated in 1998 was in primary healthcare, where the previous government's GP fundholding scheme was rapidly replaced with new primary care groups (PCGs). These local PCGs were to provide primary care and public health services for a smaller population (100,000 on average, although this varied as they were supposed to incorporate what were termed 'natural communities' i.e., pre-existing local boroughs) than that of the pre-existing local health

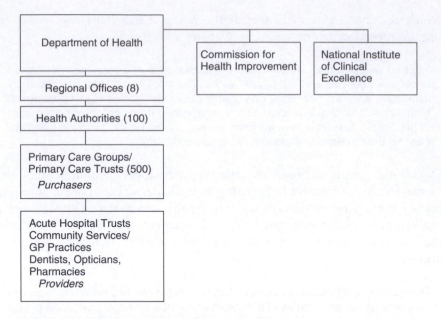

Figure 4.3 The 1998 organisational structure of the NHS

authorities, but initially were to operate under their auspices. The intention was that PCGs would gradually take on a greater range of strategic planning and local commissioning responsibilities, and eventually become primary care trusts (PCTs), doing away with the need for the local health authorities. This process was speeded up by the Department of Health, and by 2004 there were some 300 PCTs in existence. Although the PCTs replaced the system of GP fundholding, this did not represent a return to a unitary system of primary healthcare delivery. On the contrary, the new PCTs represented a structural endorsement and expansion of GP commissioning of secondary care, maintaining the purchaser–provider split. It should be noted here that with its newly devolved powers, the Scottish parliament decided to return to a unitary provider system in primary care (see next section for more details of the Health service arrangements in Scotland and Northern Ireland).

The New Labour government's promotion of what they termed 'supply-led' reforms to the structure of the NHS in England and Wales and began to take shape in its second term of office (2001–2005), in effect constituted an expansion of the internal market in healthcare. The government promoted the benefits of market 'incentives' but not market 'competition' (a term which was eschewed given its associations with the fragmentation of services that occurred within the Conservative government's internal market) between a range of healthcare providers. In its third term of government (2005–), the New Labour government has deepened these

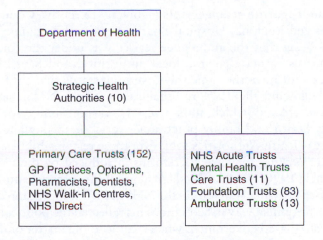

Figure 4.4 The organisational structure of the NHS in 2008

supply-side reforms of the structure of the NHS. These changes have seen the expansion of 'foundation hospital trusts' (at the beginning of 2008 there were 88 such trusts in existence). These are acute hospitals and mental health trusts that have passed a series of performance tests (of financial and organisational competence) enabling them to formally operate as independent providers of secondary care, as well as a much wider role for independent sector providers in secondary, primary and long-term care.

In 2004, local health authorities and Regional offices were abolished, replaced by the PCTs which now acted as incipient local health authorities operating from a primary care base. However, in late 2006, the number of PCTs was cut in half (down to 152), justified on the grounds that this would facilitate a closer relationship between health, social care and emergency services. In 2002, 28 Strategic Health Authorities (SHAs) had been created to act as a key link between the Department of Health and the NHS, monitoring the local commissioning process, as well as the quality and performance of local services. Yet, by 2006, these were reduced to ten larger SHAs, which, it was said, would improve efficiency. These changes in the organisational structure are set out in Figure 4.4.

THE NHS IN SCOTLAND, WALES AND NORTHERN IRELAND

From its inception in 1948, differences in the organisational structures of the NHS have existed within Scotland, although until devolution in 1997 these differences were not fundamental ones. Up until 1974, Scotland had the same tripartite arrangements involving 'Executive Councils', Local Authorities and Regional Hospital Boards as existed England. The minor differences being that the ambulance service was under the control of the hospital boards rather than the local authorities, and Scottish teaching hospitals did not have the same self-governing status that they enjoyed in England. Following the 1974 re-organisation of the NHS, new hospital boards were created which took over the responsibility for hospitals, community health and family practitioner services; in England the newly created Area Health Authorities took over these responsibilities. The internal market *Working for Patients* reforms introduced by the Conservative government in 1990, which created GP fundholding practices and instigated the purchaser-provider split within the NHS in England, was introduced in a much more piecemeal way in Scotland. This reflected the political caution of a Westminster-based government when it came to the matter of introducing its welfare state reforms within Scotland.

When New Labour came to office in 1997, it was on the basis of an electoral commitment to devolution for Scotland. The new Scottish Parliament was given legislative powers, which included command over Scottish health services. The Scottish Parliament subsequently rejected the expansion of the internal market seen in England, although parallel agencies to NICE and CHI were established. In Scotland, primary care and secondary care became the responsibility of new unified local NHS health boards with a primary responsibility for reducing inequalities and improving health; the Scottish *NHS Plan* (Scottish Executive, 2000) having prioritised the primary prevention of disease and health promotion initiatives over waiting times. One fundamental difference with the NHS in England was the decision to implement the recommendations of the Royal Commission on Long-term Care (Sutherland Commission, 1999), that all personal care carried out in residential and nursing homes be publicly funded rather than means-tested (the issues surrounding who should pay for long-term social and medical care of those with disabilities and dependencies is discussed in detail in Chapter 10).

The NHS in Wales has historically been more closely tied to the developments occurring in England. However, since the creation of the Welsh Assembly in 1999 which took over direct control of health services from the Office of the Secretary of State for Wales, there has been a significant departure from the path of 'modernisation' which has led to the expansion of the role of market forces in healthcare delivery within England. The decision was taken not to develop Primary Care Trusts, and instead Local Health Groups (LHGs), later replaced by Local Health Boards (LHBs), were created. Whilst these local primary care groups had a commissioning role like that of the PCTs, the focus was on building strong links with local government and with voluntary agencies rather than developing an internal market that enabled the private sector to play a bigger role in provision. The Welsh *NHS Plan* (National Assembly for Wales, 2001) unlike its English equivalent, was much more focused on public health and addressing inequalities in health, and much less concerned with reducing waiting times for secondary care. Nevertheless, the fact that the Welsh assembly lacks any of the powers that have now been devolved from Westminster to the Scottish Parliament has meant that, for example, Wales has not been able to publicly fund long-term care as has happened in Scotland.

In Northern Ireland, the NHS took on a rather different form than on the mainland, largely because of its self-governing status (suspended in 1972 as a consequence of the widening violence associated with the civil rights conflict). Post-1972, the NHS in Northern Ireland was reorganised so that responsibility for health care and social services was combined and managed by four geographically-based Health and Social Services Boards. The Conservative government internal market reforms were rolled out over a much longer period in Northern Ireland at least partly because of the complexities of the political situation, and for this reason the effects of the internal market have been longer lasting than elsewhere in Britain. The incoming New Labour government devolved powers to a new Northern Ireland Assembly following the 'Good Friday Agreement' in 1998, but following the suspension of its powers in 2002 there were delays in abolishing GP fundholding and replacing them with new primary care commissioning bodies. Since 2007, control has passed back to the Northern Ireland Assembly and a process of consultation around the re-structuring of services was begun in 2008 (DHSSPS, 2008).

In summary, following the process of the devolution of power from Westminster to the new authorities in Scotland, Wales and Northern Ireland, what has emerged is an increasing divergence from the 'modernisation' model being implemented within the NHS in England (Adams and Schmuecker, 2006). There has been a much greater focus, as represented in the health funding allocations in all three countries, on public health than upon secondary hospital-based care. This prioritisation largely reflects a political commitment to addressing the higher incidence of preventable chronic illness and a lower aggregate life expectancy for both men and women than exists in England.

SUMMARY

The purpose of this chapter has been to describe changes that have occurred in the organisational structure of the NHS since its inception in 1948. In the following chapters, there will be a detailed discussion of the process of structural and organisational reform in healthcare that have occurred since the early 1990s. But what needs to be taken from this chapter is that the debate over state funding and provision of universal healthcare was, is, and probably always will be, contentious because the demands on the system increase all the time and are most certainly not finite. The healthcare system therefore constantly has to adapt and respond to these demands, hence the history of organisational reforms that were described in this chapter, designed to improve the performance and efficiency of that system. Ultimately, however, the level of funding of healthcare is a policy issue in the largest sense of the term.

The discussion of the impact of the changes to the organisational structure of the NHS introduced by the New Labour government has been confined in this chapter to a description and setting out of organisational charts and brief comments about the expansion of the internal market first introduced during the period of the Conservative government. The proceeding chapters of the book will discuss in detail how the structural and organisational changes introduced during a decade of New Labour government health policy initiatives have played out in terms of improving the performance of the healthcare system as a whole, the consequences of widening the role of the private market within the NHS, and the ways in which they have attempted to tackle the ever-expanding demand for long-term social care services.

FURTHER READING

Beveridge, W. (1942) *Social Insurance and Allied Services*. London: HMSO.

Paton, C. (2006) *New Labour's State of Health; Political Economy, Public Policy and the NHS*. Aldershot: Ashgate.

Webster, C. (2002) *The National Health Service: a Political History* (2nd Edn). Oxford: Oxford University Press.

5 THE SYSTEM OF HEALTHCARE FUNDING IN THE UK

INTRODUCTION

The organisational transformation of the NHS has occurred against the backdrop of an increasing demand for health services arising from demographic shifts in the population and higher public expectations. Since 2002, the response of the New Labour government has been to significantly increase public spending on healthcare services in real-terms in order to meet its commitment to achieving the average spending on healthcare (measured as a proportion of GDP) of the original members of the EU. By 2007–08, annual spending on the NHS will be 40 percent higher in real-terms than it was five years earlier. At this point, the organisational and structural changes in the system of healthcare instigated in the 'modernisation' programme are expected to have achieved an improved 'performance' from the NHS in delivering high-quality 'value-for-money' services, obviating the need for further massive injections of cash. From 2008 onwards, real growth in healthcare spending is expected to be just 1–1.5 percent per annum (HM Treasury, 2004). This position assumes that public spending on the service can be managed without the need to resort to reductions or 'cuts' in the level of service, despite the fact that demand for high quality health services will continue to increase over the next decade.

FUNDING THE POST-WAR NHS

Since the ending of the Second World War, healthcare provision in Britain has been predominantly provided and funded by the state, primarily through general taxation. The NHS is partly funded through National Insurance contributions from employers and employees, although this source of funding only constitutes about one-eighth of the total NHS budget. The origins of National Insurance (NI) system lie in the early attempts to widen healthcare provision to the working classes at the beginning of the twentieth century (discussed in Chapter 4), and preceded the establishment of the NHS. The NI system is not however a system of social insurance of the type that predominates within most EU countries (a detailed discussion of funding systems found within EU healthcare systems is set out in Chapter 6 below).

State expenditure on the NHS in the 1950s and 1960s represented approximately 10 percent of all public spending (including education, defence, social services, etc.), however by the end of the 1990s this proportion had risen to 16 percent. Expenditure on the NHS has increased steadily since 1948 in order to meet the increasing demands and costs faced by the health service; this is illustrated in Figure 5.1.

There are three major factors implicated in the increasing costs of healthcare delivery which have resulted in this steady rise in spending as a proportion of GDP since 1949. These are the demographic shift that has led

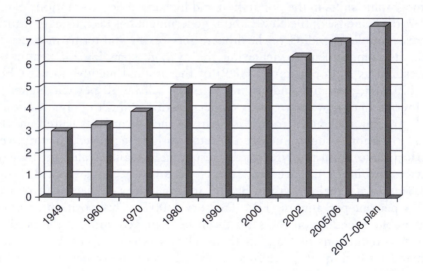

Figure 5.1 Total public expenditure on healthcare in the UK as a percentage of GDP
Sources: OECD (2005); HM Treasury (2004).

to elderly people now constituting a greater proportion of in the population; costs associated with an expanding and more skilled workforce; and the expenditure 'push' of new innovations in medical technology, the major element of which is the cost of pharmaceuticals. These three factors are intertwined with ever-increasing public expectations of the health service. One example of this process would be the demand, fuelled by the claims of the pharmaceutical companies for their new products, that there should be a drug available for every condition. Significantly, all of these factors are largely outside of the day-to-day control of the Department of Health, with the consequence that, since the inception of the NHS the costs of providing a needs-based service have consistently been underestimated by governments of all political persuasions.

A key assumption that underpinned the establishment of the NHS in 1948, and which very quickly turned out to be a naïve one, was that there was a fixed amount of illness in society. It was assumed that if sufficient resources were provided 'free at the point of consumption' then costs would gradually reduce as people became healthier. The initial high cost of funding the NHS (it exceeded its budget by almost 40 percent in its first few years) was seen as justifiable because of the unmet need that had accumulated as a consequence of the pre-war situation, when the majority of the population were not able to access appropriate health services. There was also the need to make good the chronic under-funding of the health services that had been provided by the private and voluntary sector, as well as local government. To take just two items, by 1953, 26 million pairs of glasses and 6 million sets of false teeth had been provided free of charge. Although much of this initial expenditure was a one-off spend, what was not justifiable as Lowe has argued, was the failure of the Ministry of Health's inability to '... devise a sound financial and administrative structure for future expenditure decisions' (Lowe, 1993: 175). This example of a 'non-decision' was to have long-lasting consequences for spending and budget control within the NHS. Yet another early decision also had important implications for central control over expenditure. This was the devolution of control over clinical spending to the medical profession. The subsequent later attempts to regain this control over health spending decisions through a process of regulating the activities of the medical profession, is explored in detail in Chapter 7.

By the mid-1970s, Britain was in the position of having one of the highest rates of public expenditure and direct taxation, yet one of the lowest rates of economic growth of all the modern industrialised Western economies. The Conservative Party then in opposition and now led by Margaret Thatcher had, following its adoption of what was then known as the 'new right' political ideology, explicitly cited the 'Keynesian-Beveridgean post-war settlement' for 'excessive' state spending. This 'command-and-control' state as it was termed was explicitly blamed for the country's economic decline in the 1970s. However, when the Conservative government came to power in 1979 on the back of an electoral pledge to reduce overall public spending and cut income tax, it found itself in the difficult position of trying to maintain public confidence in an 'under-funded' health service. Although spending levels were maintained during the eighteen years of Conservative governments, the public began to gradually lose confidence that the NHS was 'safe in the Conservative government's hands', to paraphrase Margaret Thatcher herself.

By the late 1980s, despite an increase in resources going to healthcare as represented by its share of total public expenditure rising from 11.8 percent in 1950 to 14.7 percent in 1988, there was an ever widening gap between state expenditure on the NHS and the funding that was needed to meet the increasing demand for health services. This under-funding of public services reflected wider problems within the economy. In 1983, unemployment had peaked at over 3 million people (based on official statistics; the real figure was almost certainly much higher) or over 12 percent of the working population, and even by 1988 continued to remain at a post-war high of over 8 percent. As the funding of the NHS had historically been closely tied to the performance of the economy (primarily funded out of general taxation), the economic recession which resulted in reduced tax revenue (fewer able to make tax contributions and an increasing demand on expenditure in the form of unemployment benefit and other benefits) had a direct impact upon the NHS budget.

The growth rate for health spending in the five-year period up to 1987, adjusted to take account of the inflationary costs faced by the health service, was running at less than 1 percent each year. This was lower even than the Department of Health's own estimate that at least a 2 percent per year increase in spending was required to keep pace with the costs of new medical technology, the demands associated with changing demographics and disease patterns, as well the demands of new forms of service delivery (Baggott, 2004: 134). By 1987, the cumulative effect of this under-funding had led to the cancelling of non-urgent admissions, the closing of hospital wards and the freezing of staff vacancies. In protest, hospital workers including nurses and doctors, took part in industrial action to highlight the effects of 'The Cuts' (as they became widely known and understood) were having on patient care. It was in response to this political crisis that the Conservative Prime Minister, Margaret Thatcher, initiated a far-reaching review (which notably excluded representatives of the medical and nursing professions) of the future of the NHS which ultimately led to the *Working for Patients* 'internal market' reforms (described in Chapter 4), presented as a 'solution' to the perennial problem of funding the NHS.

THE FINANCIAL IMPACT OF THE PURCHASER–PROVIDER SPLIT IN THE NHS

Whether the Conservative's internal market improved the overall efficiency of the health service is subject to dispute. This reflects a debate about the validity and accuracy of the measures of cost-efficiency that were deployed, the huge administrative costs that were incurred (employing more managerial staff, creating new costing and payment systems from scratch) which were glossed over by the Department of Health at the time, and the focus on acute services to the detriment of primary and preventive care service. Certainly, there was an over-reliance on generating efficiencies within an under-funded NHS. Real increases in expenditure following the introduction of the internal market did not keep pace with the increase in spending arising from 'demographic pull and technological push' (Powell, 1997: 127). This situation was not to change until the massive injection of state funding by the New Labour government in 2002.

New Labour came into government in 1997 on the back of a commitment to address the under-funding crisis faced by the health service by raising spending year-on-year in real-terms. However, in the first two years of government, expenditure on the health service rose only slowly in line with Gordon Brown's, the Chancellor of the Exchequer, commitment to sticking with the previous governments public spending plans in order to avoid 'over-heating' the economy and so establish the Labour governments reputation for financial 'prudence'. But, following criticisms of the government that it was not getting waiting list times down as quickly as it had promised, Tony Blair, the Prime Minister, made a pledge in January 2000 on BBC Television's *David Frost Programme* to raise spending on the NHS to the average spending in the original member EU countries, (which at that time would constitute 8% of GDP). This commitment was formally reaffirmed later that year in *The NHS Plan* (DoH, 2000a). Following the publication of Derek Wanless's major review of health financing (Wanless, 2001), the Chancellor of the Exchequer, who had commissioned the review, accepted the report's main recommendations and committed the government in his 2002 budget to increasing spending on the NHS by 7.4 percent (real-terms) per year between 2002–03 and 2007–08, in order to achieve this goal of matching average EU levels of funding. However, as from April 2008, the period of increases in real spending growth came to an end, having in principle achieved its goal of bringing healthcare spending in the UK upto the EU average. The recent spending increase is illustrated in Figure 5.2 below, in terms of both the annual real-term public expenditure on health and the year-on-year changes in net expenditure in percentage terms. The dramatic nature of this increase in spending is contextualised by showing the figures for the tail-end of John Major's Conservative government (1992–97), then through the small increases in real-terms in the first two years of the new Labour government (1997–99), through to the real-term increases that will end in 2008.

Despite the significant real-terms increase in public expenditure on the NHS since 2002, many NHS Trusts began to experience financial problems. On aggregate, NHS trusts overspent by more than £1.2 billion in 2005–06, a process that continued in 2006–07. This led to job cuts and the closure of hospital beds and units in hospitals around the country. An understandable polarisation in the debate surrounding the causes of this financial crisis soon emerged, with health service trade unions and professional associations arguing that this represented a crisis of national under-funding of 'hands-on' patient services in the face of demands that the government had failed to anticipate. The NHS Executive and Department of Health argued that overspending reflected local management deficiencies in financial planning not central government under-funding. The financial deficiencies of local Trusts included a failure to anticipate the consequences of the significant pay increases awarded to all health service staff. This followed

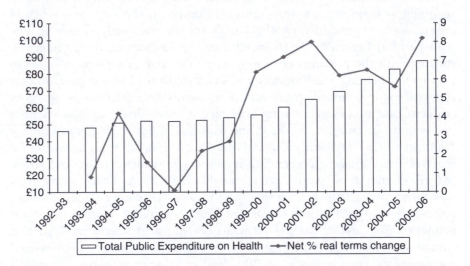

Figure 5.2 Public expenditure on NHS in the UK in real-terms[1] (£ billion), and the change in net expenditure in real-terms[2] (%) 1992–93 to 2005–06
Sources: HM Treasury (2006); DoH (1999; 2001a; 2004a; 2006a).
Notes
(1) Real-term figures are the HM Treasury cash figures adjusted to 2004–05 price levels using GDP deflators.
(2) Actual year-end position in cash terms (Outurn) percentage change in net revenue, based on Department of Health annual expenditure figures.

the implementation of the new pay structures and terms and conditions set out in the *Agenda for Change* national agreement with the staff trade unions and professional bodies (DoH, 2004b).

Recent developments relating to changes in the funding and financial arrangements within provider trusts have contributed to this crisis. In early 2006, the Department of Health introduced new financial accounting rules designed to strengthen incentives for trusts to improve productivity. Some providers were now required to reduce their unit costs on average by 4–5 percent, and some a lot higher in order to achieve financial balance by the end of the financial year (DoH, 2006b). Many trusts subsequently found that they could not 'trade their way out of deficits' because the purchasing PCTs were no longer given the funds from central government to pay for extra healthcare services provided by the trusts. The second development was the introduction of the 'Payment by Results' (PbR) system in 2005. The background to this organisational reform is discussed in detail in Chapter 9, but what appears to have emerged early on in the implementation of this system is that the tariffs or fixed payments that have been set for particular healthcare procedures have some unintended effects. Trusts were forced to close down services that appeared to be making 'losses' only because the tariffs themselves have been poorly designed and set at too low a level (Palmer, 2006: 25).

The point that needs to be made about these recent financial reforms is that they have been introduced by central government to ensure the smooth operation of the internal market in healthcare. However, those health policy analysts who take an essentially pro-market perspective, have drawn the conclusion that the internal market reforms have not gone far enough and quickly enough when they see provider trusts finding themselves in deficit. That is, the crisis has arisen because the rapid growth in NHS funding post-2002 occurred prior to putting in place; '... adequate levers to manage demand and induce improvements in provider productivity' (Palmer, 2006: 26). Those health policy analysts who take the opposite view, and who argue that the market reforms have gone too far in the NHS, see the expansion of the internal market in healthcare as the primary cause of the financial crisis. The argument that is made is that the creation of a 'supplier market' in the NHS has served to prevent the massive increases in NHS funding since 2002 being fed into improved patient services. According to Julian Tudor-Hart, the NHS has now been transformed:

> ... into a management agency commissioning care through competing contractors investing for profit. It argues that these policies have imposed business methods and ethics akin to the rest of commercial society. This policy necessarily incurs higher administrative cost, obvious from the rising percentage of total spending

on healthcare devoted to administration, transactions, legal support and profit for contractors. In the pre-reform NHS this amounted to less than 6 percent, increasing to 12 per cent by 2004, and approaching 20 per cent today. In the United States, where they use a comparable model to that favoured by the current management consensus, administrative costs account for, on average, over 30 percent of total costs (Tudor-Hart, 2006: 8).

ACTIVITY

Some health policy commentators have claimed that the NHS is transforming itself from a public service into the 'industrial' model of healthcare provision found in the USA that is generally referred to as 'Managed Care' (Tudor-Hart, 2006: 15). Managed Care is characterised by a wresting of control over healthcare resources and planning from care professionals and placed in the hands of corporations driven by market incentives, so that 'unprofitable' patients, such as those requiring long-term care or those who are more at risk of ill-health lose out because of their materially disadvantageous position in society.

Identify the elements of the recent reforms within the NHS that may support (or deny) such an assertion.

THE ROLE OF PRIVATE FINANCE IN THE NHS

In 2005, spending on the NHS as a publicly funded healthcare service represented 83 percent (in 1949, the figure was 88 percent) of total healthcare expenditure in the UK, with the remaining 17 percent being privately financed. From these figures it is apparent that the private market sector continues to be a comparatively minor player in healthcare provision in the UK compared with countries such as the USA. Nevertheless, the NHS has since its foundation always been ready to draw upon and encourage the use of private capital in service provision. Private 'pay beds' have always been available to purchase in NHS hospitals, particularly in the London Teaching hospitals, which are conveniently located near the private practices of consultants in central London. These pay beds served as an additional source of cash to many hospital-based consultants and to the hospitals themselves. However, the number of pay beds was always small and largely limited to London hospitals. The real increase in the scale of the private sector's contribution to NHS activity occurred in the mid-1980s when 'privatisation' of NHS services became the official policy of the then Conservative government. Hospital support services such as cleaning, meal services and maintenance were 'contracted out' to the private market as they were no longer seen to be 'core' NHS activities (one of the consequences of this development has been a decline in the standard of cleaning which may have contributed to the rise of MRSA infections). Also, from this period on there was a significant expansion of the involvement of the private sector in key sectors of health and social care provision. These include a large bulk of long-term residential and nursing home care (discussed in detail in Chapter 10), all routine optical services and the majority of dental care. In relation to dentistry, the NHS has essentially has become a residual service providing treatment to children and those adults unable to afford the full cost.

Although the effective privatisation of many NHS services in the 1980s and 1990s changed the complexion of the health service, even these changes did not match the levels of private capital that have permeated into the NHS since 1998, following New Labour's 'modernisation' strategy. Two policy developments in particular can be identified as bringing about this shift towards a dependency on private capital investment. First, the building of the 'supplier market' in service provision that followed the transfer of over 80 percent of the NHS budget to PCTs in order to facilitate the process of local commissioning (retaining the purchaser–provider split of the internal market) of services (described in detail in Chapter 9). The second key development was the expansion of the Private Finance Initiative (PFI) instigated by the previous Conservative government. Since 2000 this development has subsequently become known as 'Public–Private Partnerships' (PPP).

The PFI had been conceived by the Conservative government in the early 1990s, partly in response to the recession in the building industry (which many leading Conservative politicians had close ties to). Allyson Pollock, in her highly acclaimed critical book *NHS Plc*, has described the PFI (or PPP) scheme as it operates within the NHS as follows:

'Special purpose vehicles' or SPV's ... (consisting of) consortia of construction companies, facilities management companies and banks, would raise money by issuing shares and borrowing, to build, own and operate public service premises such as hospitals. Hospital trusts would lease the buildings, complete with maintenance and other support staff, under contracts lasting twenty-five to thirty years or even more. As well as offering rich returns to the private sector the PFI was presented as a way of getting new buildings without raising taxes, at least in the short run .... the public would still be paying for the hospitals, but payment would be deferred, like hire purchase but minus the purchase, since when a PFI hospital contract comes to an end the land and buildings will in most cases still belong to the private owners, not the NHS (Pollock, 2004: 53).

Here, Pollock is describing a set of processes that she argues amount to the 'progressive dismantling and privatisation' of the NHS (2004: 2). Capital spending on the building of new hospitals and the provision of primary care facilities had been minimal since the 1980s, indeed between 1980 and 1997 only seven NHS capital schemes of any kind costing more than £25 million were completed (Gaffney et al., 1999: 48). But with the embracing of the PFI, the New Labour government was able to announce in 2002 that 34 PFI hospital projects had been completed or the contracts signed for, with a further 55 major hospital schemes in the pipeline (DoH, 2002). Since 2002, although the PFI has been strongly criticised for not delivering value-for-money in the long term, it remains the primary method for the delivery of new NHS capital projects. Since 2004, the involvement of private finance in primary care has also expanded with the development of the Local Improvement Finance Trusts (LIFTs), private Limited Companies who are created to deliver PFI-type contracts at a local level to build primary and community care facilities. This development has resulted in GPs having to increasingly lease their premises from private corporations when expanding their facilities. In 2007, the Department of Health announced yet another new PFI initiative (DoH, 2007e) for delivering social care facilities in the community in line with the principles of moving long-term care away from hospitals nearer to people's homes as set out in the social care White Paper, *Our Health, Our Care, Our Say* (DoH, 2006c).

In summary, PFI is more expensive than public financing of capital projects (because the NHS does not need to borrow money from banks at a commercial rate), and the costs of paying for these new buildings come out of current operating revenues, giving little flexibility to meet rising demand. PFI schemes lock hospital trusts into paying for buildings over several decades when the original requirement for these buildings may well have changed as the health needs of the population change. This process inevitably distorts the focus of hospitals' planning and investing to meet local health needs because of the requirement to service the repayments to private PFI companies. In a very real way, the NHS as a national system of state healthcare provision is now being extensively penetrated by private capital. For, in addition to the supply market in healthcare provision and PFI building programmes, the National Programme for IT (NPfIT) in the NHS (the rolling out of electronic patient records and other information initiatives) is also heavily dependent on private finance and expertise. As Pollock has described it; '… very soon every part of (the NHS) will have been "unbundled" and commodified' (Pollock, 2004: 214). Whilst this quotation may be somewhat overstating the case, the impact of the processes described in this quote, are absolutely fundamental for the future of the NHS as we have known it for sixty years.

ACTIVITY

This Activity asks you to think about the levels of funding that would be required to meet and sustain healthcare needs in the UK today. Attempt to answer the following question, Should the government place a ceiling on state funding of health care services beyond which individuals should make private arrangements to meet their health costs? – focus on (a) the practical difficulties involved (b) whether setting a ceiling on state expenditure undermines the founding principles of the NHS.

SUMMARY

Although separated for the purposes of simplifying the historical processes involved, the chapters on healthcare structures and on healthcare funding imply a distinction between the organisation and funding of healthcare which in practice is an artificial one. The organisational and funding structures of the NHS have been, and always will be, inextricably linked in practice. Nevertheless, the ongoing development of the internal market which organisationally separates the purchasers or 'commissioners' and the providers of health services, together with the increasing penetration of the NHS by private capital, may (ironically) have had the effect of clouding the impact of the very real increases in public expenditure on healthcare that have occurred. This is ironic in the sense that the building of new financial arrangements within the NHS to facilitate the development of the supplier market in healthcare (facilitating private and voluntary organisations to compete for service contracts) has brought with it its own set of problems leading to a public perception that the NHS is in financial 'crisis.'

FURTHER READING

Pollock, A. (2004) *NHS plc*. London: Verso.
Wanless, D. (2002) *Securing our Future Health: Taking a Long-term View – Final Report*. London: HM Treasury.

6 A COMPARATIVE ANALYSIS OF EUROPEAN HEALTHCARE SYSTEMS: CHANGING DEMANDS, COMMON SOLUTIONS?

CHAPTER CONTENTS

- Introduction
- An introduction to comparative health and social policy analysis
- State intervention in healthcare: the formation of European healthcare systems
- The changing demands upon European healthcare systems
- Comparing European healthcare systems across three dimensions – finance, provision, and regulation
- Is there a process of convergence between European healthcare systems?
- Summary

INTRODUCTION

Studying the British National Health Service in isolation from developments in healthcare systems in other similarly developed countries can all too easily lead to an overestimating of the uniqueness of the problems faced by the NHS in delivering an effective and efficient health service. In this chapter, the changing and increasing healthcare demands experienced by most developed countries (note that membership of the Organisation of Economic Co-operation and Development is used here as shorthand for a country that could also be described as 'developed'; it also reflects the ready availability of comparable statistics produced by the OECD), together with the discernable trends in the health policy responses of these countries to these demands will be assessed in order to contextualise the process of organisational change occurring within the United Kingdom's NHS. The analysis of these developments will draw upon the previous discussion of the role of the state (in Chapter 2) in relation to the process of change now occurring within national healthcare systems within the European Union.

The primary focus of this chapter is a comparative analysis of healthcare systems within the European Union rather than all 30 member countries of the OECD. Although the different European national healthcare systems were historically developed at different times reflecting distinct political, social and cultural priorities, today they all face the very similar challenges of having an ageing population with all its attendant needs, and a predominant reliance on state funding and provision of services. By contrast, the healthcare system(s) that exist within the USA, and to some extent in Australasia, face very different sorts of challenges that would require a comparative analysis of much longer length than could be accommodated within this general text.

AN INTRODUCTION TO COMPARATIVE HEALTH AND SOCIAL POLICY ANALYSIS

International comparisons of healthcare systems are difficult to make for a number of reasons. Firstly, the constituents of healthcare provision may differ across countries. This in part reflects the ways in which the health and social care 'divide' is defined (see Chapter 10 for a detailed discussion of this 'divide' in the UK), as well as where the boundary between 'formal' and 'informal' care is drawn. Secondly, national healthcare system data are frequently not directly comparable. For example British GPs are formally independent contractors of primary care services to the NHS, but does that make them private sector employees as they would be in some EU countries? Finally, there will always be the potential for false or misinformed assumptions to be drawn when attempting to compare countries with different social, demographic, economic and political structures. There are then a range of potentially compounding methodological pitfalls that need to be avoided in generating comparable data sensitive to the differing cultural and political contexts of cross-national health policy. Hence, the increasingly influential view of comparative social and health policy analysis is that it does not constitute a distinct and substantive area of academic study in and of itself. Rather, its distinctive contribution lies in its employment as a methodological strategy used to illuminate cross-national policy questions and hypotheses (Higgins, 1986: 24).

The emphasis on the convergence of health and welfare systems in modern states, as measured primarily by expenditure as a proportion of GNP that once dominated comparative policy analysis, is increasingly being superseded by forms of analyses that seek to explain both qualitative as well as quantitative differences in healthcare systems. In large comparative policy studies of countries (the regular OECD Health Data survey would be one such example) which draw upon the statistical analysis of a relatively limited number of quantitative variables such as GNP, public sector proportions of social spending and mortality rates or income inequality, individual countries as distinct socio-politico-cultural entities tend to disappear. In contrast, comparative studies that look at just a limited number of countries tend to treat them as 'multi-dimensional backgrounds' for comparing the content of, or change within particular social and health policy programmes. The distinctiveness of this type of comparative research is that it conceptualises national social and health policies (which in structure may superficially look similar in a number of countries) as embedded within distinct political, social and ideological contexts, which in turn impinge on the shape and impact of these policies (Clasen, 2004: 94–95).

It is possible to identify two broad 'ideal-type' healthcare systems (National Health service models and Social Insurance models), based upon the examination of the three dimensions of healthcare (finance, provision, and regulation) as they apply to actual healthcare systems (Figure 6.1). The use of these ideal-types does need to be tempered with the understanding that they reflect only a generalised analysis of healthcare systems, and that national political, economic, and cultural priorities mean that change within healthcare systems is an ongoing process. The playing out of these structural and organisational changes at the national level may mean that

Ideal-type	Financing	Provision	Regulation	Examples
National Health Service model	Direct (income) and indirect forms (consumption) of public taxation	Public	Top-down, command-and-control by the state bureaucracy	UK, Denmark, Sweden, Finland, Italy (since 1978), Spain (since 1986)
Social Insurance model	Public contributions based on income	Private and public providers	Corporatist model of collective bargaining between providers and purchasers	France, Germany, Austria, Belgium, Netherlands

Figure 6.1 Two main ideal-types of EU Healthcare systems

fewer countries may in the future fit the ideal-type, weakening the heuristic usefulness of the typology. On the other hand, systems may be converging in terms of their key features (this issue is discussed below), thus strengthening the usefulness of the ideal-type.

STATE INTERVENTION IN HEALTHCARE: THE FORMATION OF EUROPEAN HEALTHCARE SYSTEMS

As Freeman (2000a) has noted:

> (M)ore or less casually used, the notion of *health system* tends to reinforce understandings of it in functional terms. But the issue here is not that different modes of organisation make systems more or less expensive or efficient, though that is undoubtedly important, but that they have different political implications. One way of addressing these is by foregrounding the state (Freeman, 2000a: 8) emphasis in original

This section will examine the formation of healthcare systems within Western Europe and seek to explain why the differences that exist between these organisational forms reflect the different political and cultural role historically played by the state within these different countries.

EU member states do not all spend similar proportions of their Gross Domestic Product (GDP) on healthcare. The East European states, for example, which joined the expanded EU in 2004, started from a much lower baseline in terms of per capita spending and countries such as Spain, Greece and Portugal have the political legacy of repressive regimes which largely ignored the health and welfare needs of their citizens. However, what is common to nearly all these European countries (as represented in Figure 6.2) is that the primary source of this healthcare funding comes through the public sector (on average between 70–80 percent among EU member-states); with the private market having a much smaller role to play than in the USA, for example.

A dominant contemporary view, widely found across Western Europe countries, conceives the finance and provision of healthcare as being essentially a 'public service' rather than a 'private concern'. This popular view can be said to reflect the original political and ideological justification for the creation of welfare states in post-war Europe. Such 'planner states' (an independent national public power separate from profit and party politics – Webster, 2002) were seen as acting in the 'national interest' in separating the provision of services to meet the educational, welfare and health needs of its citizenry from the partisan interests of

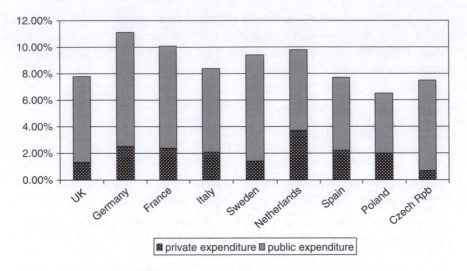

Figure 6.2 Total expenditure on healthcare – public sector and private market share of spending: percentage share of GDP by selected countries 2003 (OECD, 2005)

private companies. As a representative of this model of the progressive expansion of citizenship rights designed to limit the effects of class disadvantage (including inequalities in health outcome), the British NHS would be seen as a public service based not on profit or private gain but on a 'gift economy' (voluntary blood donation being a prime example of this process as described in Richard Titmuss's [1970a] classic book on the subject). However, one caveat that does need to be added is that, in the case of the Eastern European countries that joined the EU in 2004, the transition from forms of state socialism to liberal democracy meant that relative equality and the provision of universal public services were the starting points (in the sense that these formally existed under the previous communist regimes) rather than the end goal of change in the relationship between the state and citizen (Watson, 2004).

Despite the apparently similar interventionary role now played by EU states in healthcare, the path towards establishing these systems has not been a uniform one, reflecting their different political, economic, and cultural histories. In Chapter 2, the essentially contested role of the modern state was explored at length (and diagrammatically represented in Figure 2.1). The intention here is not to reiterate these different theoretical positions, rather the concern is to say something about the broad historical and economic factors that led to what has been described as the '*étatisation*' (widening state involvement) of health and healthcare in Europe (Freeman, 2000a: 14); not withstanding the point made above concerning the different paths of development that have been followed by nation states during this process.

There are a number of examples of state intervention in health prior to the beginning of the twentieth century, such as the regulation of institutional care, the accreditation of healthcare professions, and notably the introduction of public health legislation and enforcement in the mid-nineteenth century. However, most of the texts that examine the history of the development of the role of state regard the introduction of statutory health insurance schemes for the population (or at least the skilled male working-class part of the population) as the point at which the national state first becomes inextricably involved in healthcare provision. The first substantive example of a public, compulsory system of health insurance was in nineteenth-century Germany, with the enactment of the Workers Sickness Insurance Act of 1883. This was followed in Britain by the passing of the Health Insurance Act in 1911, whilst compulsory insurance was only introduced for all employees in France as late as 1930.

The interesting feature of the development of public healthcare finance was that its first manifestations were local mutual aid sickness schemes. Generally speaking these were examples of skilled manual workers coming together to secure some degree of security from the consequences of falling sick and being unable to work. These collectivist forms of provision later became models for state compulsory insurance schemes. Freeman (2000a: 17) has argued that this connection between social insurance schemes and industrial labour reflects the interrelated processes of industrialisation and democratisation that were emergent towards the end of the nineteenth century. These democratic processes reflected not only the extension of the franchise to adult males across Western Europe, but also the pressure then being applied to political systems as greater numbers of workers became organised within trade unions, which articulated their demands for greater job security and welfare rights.

All these factors certainly played an important role in the foundation of what might be termed the first 'healthcare state' in Germany in the 1880s. At this time Germany was experiencing an economic boom following its unification in 1871 which accelerated an ongoing process of industrialisation and urbanisation (it had 2 million factory workers in 1867, but fifteen years later this had tripled to 6 million). These socio-economic changes led to unsafe working conditions as well as the loss of traditional forms of social protection, i.e., close-knit family and community support, in the case of sickness or injury. The social reforms instigated by the German Chancellor, Bismarck, introduced publicly mandated sickness insurance scheme, including industrial injury insurance and pensions. These reforms were introduced as an explicit political bribe in which welfare benefits were offered to promote the political allegiance of an increasingly radicalised and organised working class to the new 'Bismarckian' political and social order. This 'defensive' pattern was to be later followed in Sweden, which had a similar autocratic regime to that which existed in Germany in the late nineteenth century. Elsewhere, in those countries where parliamentary democracies had developed much earlier such as in Britain and France, state intervention in health insurance provision was slower to come about largely because the liberal market-orientated politics of these countries were more wary of state intervention (Freeman, 2000a: 20). When these countries did introduce statutory social insurance schemes in the early twentieth century these were independently (of the state) organised and managed. This best fitted the liberal political view that benefits should reflect contributions, as much as it was seen to mollify an organised working class agitating for better working conditions and an expansion of social rights.

The common pattern that emerged in relation to the development of statutory social and health insurance schemes by Western European states which were gradually extended to cover the majority of the working population, are also discernable in the process of universalising access to publicly financed and provided hospital and primary care services for the majority of the populations in Western European countries (by the 1970s). The need for national states to ensure their continuing legitimacy in the face of rising demands for an extension of the social rights of citizenship (processes that were described in detail in relation to the development of the British welfare state in Chapter 4) formed the social and political context for the development of universal healthcare services across Western European states. However, this was not a uniform process and like the development of statutory social insurance two distinct historical routes are discernable.

In France and Germany, the process was one of incremental expansion of the statutory insurance scheme to include previously excluded groups. However, this process left a legacy of healthcare complexity (resulting in comparatively high healthcare costs compared with the UK, for example), reflecting the wide diversity of insurers (covering the different social and occupational groups), providers (public, private and voluntary), as well as the involvement of local, regional and national governments which are only now being addressed through a thorough-going process of organisational reform.

In Britain, Sweden (and later Italy) the introduction of universal access to healthcare was more radical acheived, through the creation of a national (or nationalised) health service (in 1946 in Britain, 1947 in Sweden, and 1978 in Italy). This was in response to the failure of the pre-war complex mixture of voluntary, private and local government provision to effectively, efficiently, or equitably meet the healthcare needs of the population. Significantly, these countries also had radical social democratic governments who were politically committed to universalising the pre-war partial healthcare and insurance systems as a social right of citizenship. A third factor was the determination of the state in Britain and Sweden to override (although concessions were made) the sectional interests of the medical profession who were opposed to what they perceived as the extension of state control over their traditional autonomy. However, in practice, this autonomy was enhanced by their position of dominance within these national healthcare systems (a process discussed in detail in relation to the UK in Chapter 7). Whereas the instability of the post-war governments in France (up until the 1960s) enabled the medical profession to in effect exercise a veto over any radical reform of the healthcare system.

The most direct consequence of the introduction of the post-war state health insurance schemes for the vast majority of the population was to unleash the pent-up demand for healthcare within most Western European countries. This demand was met with an expansion of supply in the form of hospital-building programmes and, in the case of those countries with national health services such as Britain and Sweden, the effective 'nationalisation' or taking into state ownership or control the patchwork of voluntary, local authority and private hospitals. Up until the late 1970s in most EU countries, state involvement in the day-to-day regulation of healthcare delivery was restricted for the most part to matters of finance, concerned with ways for paying for treatment and investment in health facilities. Central governments were largely unconcerned with the forms of care being delivered within the healthcare system, this remained the preserve of doctors (Freeman, 2000a: 27). This all changed when these same European governments were faced with the consequences of a global economic downturn, with numbers of unemployed rising and tax revenues diminishing. The implications of the belated acknowledgement that there were limits to the expansion of healthcare systems began to be debated in earnest from the early 1980s. This political debate about the effective and efficient organisation of healthcare delivery ultimately led on to a wave of healthcare reform programmes (beginning in Britain in 1989 with the internal market reforms of the Conservative government). This debate was tempered by the knowledge that the healthcare systems of these European countries all faced new demands and challenges as they moved into the twenty-first century.

THE CHANGING DEMANDS UPON EUROPEAN HEALTHCARE SYSTEMS

Health spending grew faster than GDP in every OECD country (Finland being the only exception) between 1990 and 2004. It accounted for 7 percent of GDP on average across OECD countries in 1990 but reached 8.9 percent in 2004, (OECD, 2006c). This rise in the proportion of spending reflected the changing demands now experienced by healthcare systems within developed countries. Three major factors are broadly identified in the literature as being responsible for this increase in spending. These factors are, first, a changing demography marked particularly by ageing populations; second, developments in medical technologies and their associated costs; and third, the rising public expectations of healthcare services.

The demographic trend towards an increasingly ageing population is a common feature of most developed countries (see Figure 6.3). Globally, this trend is a product of two processes: a decline in fertility and increased life expectancy. Within Western societies, it is primarily the decline in fertility rates resulting both from social and biological processes which have increased the proportion of elderly within these societies. The increasing elderly population is also exacerbated by the exceptionally large age cohort known as 'baby boomers' – the generation born following the end of the Second World War. This has produced a situation where what is known as the 'dependency-ratio'[1] will increase dramatically over the next decade as the 'baby-boomer generation reaches the age of retirement (see Figure 6.4

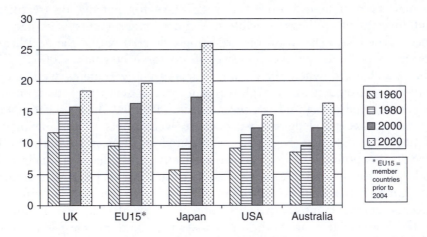

Figure 6.3   Ageing societies – population aged 65 and over, as percentage of total population of selected countries (OECD, 2006)

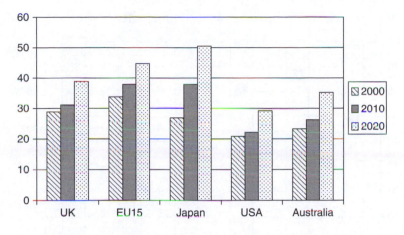

Figure 6.4 Ageing and dependency – population aged 65 and over, as percentage of total labour force in selected countries (OECD, 2006)

for a diagrammatic representation of the proportion of over 65-year-olds compared with those in the labour force). This demographic shift has the important consequence of reducing the tax base of a country, a process that has been concentrating minds amongst those involved in policy decision-making in most developed countries for some time given its implications for the public financing of social security, pensions, and healthcare.

The increase in life expectancy is also an important factor in the demand for healthcare, but within this overall trend the ageing of the elderly population itself (marked by a rising proportion of over 80-year-olds) is of particular significance. This development is important because, beyond 80 years of age, health and disability problems start to multiply with concomitant increasing demands on healthcare resources. However, it should also be noted that the increases in longevity that have occurred within Western societies have also been accompanied by an increase in the number of years of good health that are experienced post-retirement; this is a process known as 'healthy ageing' and is assessed using the measure known as 'health life expectancy.'[2]

Major health costs come at the end of life rather than being associated with longevity *per se* (OECD, 2006b). This is one reason why there is not necessarily a direct connection between healthcare spending and life expectancy within developed countries, as demonstrated in the comparative data across selected OECD countries (presented diagrammatically in Figure 6.5). The Japanese have the highest life expectancy in the OECD area, but their health spending, measured as a proportion of GDP, is far

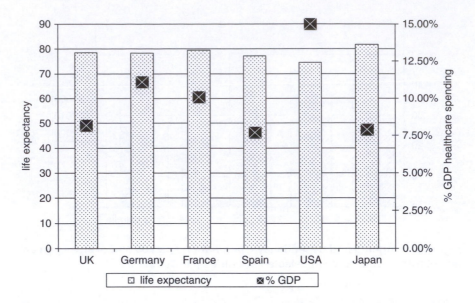

Figure 6.5 Longevity and health spending – what's the link? Life expectancy at birth in years, and health spending as a percentage of GDP by selected countries, 2003 (OECD, 2005)

from being the highest. The USA on the other hand has the highest health spending at some 15 percent of GDP, yet it has one of the lower levels of life expectancy amongst developed industrialised countries. The other factors that account for the differences in levels of healthcare spending in the major developed countries relate to the different historical forms of provision, whether predominantly public or private, as well as political and cultural factors.

The second major factor affecting the financial costs of healthcare systems is the rapid development of new medical technology. This includes not only a much wider range of pharmaceuticals, but new types of diagnostic equipment utilising new forms of imaging and genetic technology. It is difficult to be precise about the annual increase in the cost of these new medical technologies as they replace or supersede previous technology, but we can be more precise about the rising costs of pharmaceuticals which year on year constitute a growing share of health expenditure. On average, per capita spending on drugs within OECD countries has increased 5 percent per year since 1997, constituting a more than one-third increase in real terms. Most OECD countries have seen a much more rapid growth in spending on pharmaceuticals than on total health spending during this period. Spending on pharmaceuticals amongst member countries represented on average 17.5 percent of total healthcare spending

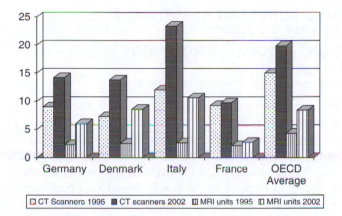

Figure 6.6 Increase in medical technology: CT scanners and MRI units per million population (OECD, 2005)

in 2003 (OECD, 2005). The increase in the expansion of medical technology is illustrated in data presented in Figure 6.6, which shows the rapid increase in the availability of highly expensive diagnostic technology such as CT scanners and MRI units in the seven years from 1995 to 2002.

The third major factor identified as bringing about new demands on healthcare systems is that of the rise in public expectations. This is a development that reflects a set of processes that go beyond the emergence of a better-informed and more articulate public demanding that there is more choice available to them as consumers of healthcare (consumerism in healthcare is discussed in detail in Chapter 9). What has been described as the 'healthcare industry' has also played its part in shaping and, indeed, creating the perceived need for new medical technologies. This healthcare industry would include the pharmaceutical companies and medical technology companies which have poured large sums of money into the research and development of new drugs and medical equipment. These companies need to generate large profits for re-investment so as to maintain their position in a highly competitive, but also highly lucrative market. The healthcare industry would also include the medical profession itself, in the sense that doctors have been trained to do the best they can for their patients within the context of what is termed the 'technological imperative.' That is, the application of new diagnostic technologies and the prescribing of the latest expensive drugs are traditionally seen by the profession to be fully justified if it can be shown that there is some benefit accruing to the patient.

COMPARING EUROPEAN HEALTHCARE SYSTEMS ACROSS THREE DIMENSIONS: FINANCE, PROVISION AND REGULATION

This section is concerned with examining both the commonalities and differences that exist between European healthcare systems. In order to achieve this goal, an analytical framework will be deployed that assesses systems on the basis of three dimensions (or 'functional processes of the health sector' – Freeman, 2000a: 1). Firstly, finance or the means by which healthcare systems are paid for; secondly, forms of healthcare provision or delivery; and third, the level at which the state intervenes to regulate the operation of the healthcare system. The relationship between these dimensions is schematically represented in Figure 6.7.

HEALTHCARE FINANCE

Within OECD countries, three distinct types of organisational arrangements used to finance the healthcare sector can be found – through the state via direct taxation, state-sponsored compulsory social insurance schemes, or forms of voluntary private insurance or individualised payment schemes. Identifying these flows of finance draws attention to the relative power of

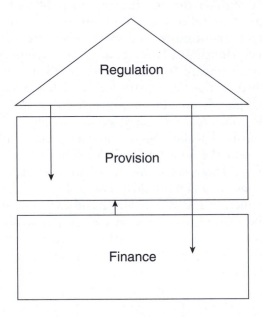

Figure 6.7   Three functional dimensions of healthcare systems

the different institutional and political actors within the healthcare sector in a given country. The most straightforward form of financing is for patients to pay doctors directly for the service that they receive. However, in most developed countries finance is managed by a third party, either the state, not-for-profit organisations, or private insurance companies. In nearly all EU member-states the primary source of financing health is public. The involvement of the state is either direct through tax-funded arrangements or indirect through the statutory social health insurance arrangements (it should also be noted that a minority of service users across these countries have private health insurance of some form). Social health insurance (SHI) provides the organising principle and preponderance of funding in half of all the pre-2004 EU states (note: the majority of the post-2004 members have gone down the SHI route), whilst the other half have tax-funded systems (with Britain having the most longstanding direct tax-based system).

SHI systems are generally recognised as having a number of core structural components (Saltman, 2004a), as follows:

1. *Contributions are independent of health risk and transparent:* Individual payment contributions to the scheme are tied to income, often to a designated ceiling, and not to the health status of the member (unlike private health insurance). The dependents of the members are automatically covered for the income-related premium. The contributions are collected separately from state taxation, meaning that premiums to the health system are transparent to the individual.

2. *Sickness pay for as purchasers:* Premiums are either collected directly through sickness funds (as in Germany, France, Austria and Switzerland) or a central state-run fund (Netherlands, Luxembourg). Both these funds are not-for-profit organisations run by an independent board but with statutory responsibilities. The funds use members premiums to fund collective contracts with healthcare providers; which can be private not-for-profit, private for-profit, or public sector.

3. *The same comprehensive benefit package for all members:* SHI coverage ranges from 63 percent of the population in the Netherlands, to 100 percent in France (where, since 2000, health insurance is no longer obtained on the basis of salary) and Switzerland. In those countries without mandatory participation, only the highest-income earners are allowed to leave the statutory system to fund their own private scheme coverage. Funding for all members is equalised with the addition of either state funds or various risk-adjustment mechanisms, because in all eight Western European countries with SHI schemes the state requires the same comprehensive health package for all.

4. *Pluralism in organisational structure:* All the SHI systems have a wide range of organisational participants. Sickness funds may vary in

their membership according to region, religion or political allegiance, and profession grouping. Virtually all hospitals, whether publicly or privately run, and primary care doctors have contracts with the sickness funds.

5. *Corporatist model of negotiations:* There is typically a 'corporatist' approach (the authority or power of each of the key organisational actors, i.e., health professions, sickness funds, unions, employers, is formally recognised or 'licensed' by the national state) to negotiating contracts. This ensures more uniformity of outcome and lower transaction costs than in a private insurance system. However, the corporatist model necessitates an open process of governance in which all the organisational actors are able to participate in the key decision-making processes.

6. *Individual choice:* Members of sickness funds can usually choose which hospital or doctor they will receive care from.

Although there is considerable diversity in structural and organisational arrangements amongst European SHI systems there are several key commonalities. First and foremost, SHI schemes have been described as a 'way of life'; '… a stable, tradition-bound social institution in which economic implications play an important role but do not exercise primary influence over decision-making' (Saltman, 2004b: 142). Secondly, SHI is central to state 'social protection' structures which forms a key pillar of civil society in these countries; the principle of social 'solidarity' being a core political principle for health and welfare provision. The third commonality relates to the complicated system of governance in which an alternative (to the state) form of control over healthcare operates through the corporatist arrangements described above and involving a range of organisational actors.

Thus the role played by the state in countries with SHI systems would appear to be of a different order than in those countries with healthcare systems funded through direct taxation. In these countries, the healthcare system is not seen as being publicly owned, in the sense that finance and provision is directly controlled by the state, rather the state is seen as the administrator and guardian of health and welfare structures (Saltman, 2004a: 5). This does not mean that the state has a weaker role in healthcare in countries with SHI systems, just a different role than in countries with direct-taxation systems. The state remains the ultimate decision-maker in relation to the determination of the range of health benefits available, the rules for contracting, determining whether there should be mandatory membership, how contributions are calculated, and the degree of discretion in decision-making enjoyed by sickness funds (Busse, Saltman and Dubois, 2004: 58).

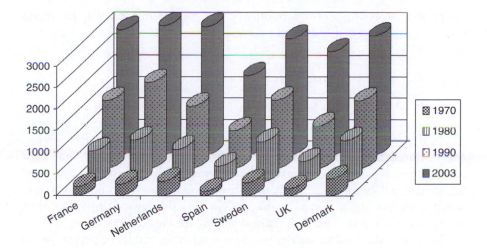

Figure 6.8 Trends in total expenditure per capita (in $ per person) 1970–2003 (OECD, 2005)

The new challenges faced by, and increased demands upon healthcare systems that are described above, have led to a significant increase in real-term healthcare spending over the past decade compared to the steady but slow growth of the previous thirty to forty years in Western European healthcare systems (see Figure 6.8). Average growth rates in the 15 countries of the EU (pre-2004) in the period 1997–2003 were 4.2 percent in real terms, and equivalent average figure of 4.3 percent holds across all OECD countries in the same period, compared to between 2 percent and 2.5 percent in the 1980s (OECD, 2005).

In countries with SHI systems, these new demands have raised important questions about the financial sustainability of the existing healthcare finance arrangements. As a consequence, the German state intervened in the late 1990s to restrict flows of funds by coupling increases in SHI premiums to increase in overall salary levels as an incentive to sickness funds to become more cost-effective. In France, an alternative approach was adopted, here the state intervened to expand the revenue base for SHI by introducing a new wealth-based tax. A number of other states have also attempted to act to restrict the growth in the above inflation rise in the cost of pharmaceuticals (described above). However, there is no overall evidence that SHI systems are less (or more) cost-effective than tax-based systems (Figueras et al., 2004). Equally, when Derek Wanless was asked by the British government in 2002 to review the future funding and organisation of the NHS, his report concluded that the evidence showed that alternative funding systems such as SHI systems; '... would not deliver a given quality of healthcare either at a lower cost to the economy or in a more equitable way (to direct taxation)' (Wanless, 2002: para 6.66).

HEALTHCARE PROVISION

The role of the state in healthcare in EU member-states extends beyond financing, whether through direct taxation or the overseeing of SHI systems, to an involvement (greater or lesser) in the provision of health services for its population. The range of service provision arrangements that exist across the EU member-states may be schematically represented along an organisational axis from a totally private market through to a universal state scheme. Points along this axis indicate the possible mix of private/public providers in the national healthcare systems (see Figure 6.9).

These provider healthcare organisations, whether public or private, have traditionally been shaped by the clinical requirements of the medical profession. A detailed analysis of the relationship between the state and the profession within the UK is the concern of the following chapter (see Chapter 7), therefore only a few outline comments will be made here. In Britain, the post-war establishment of the NHS provided the opportunity for the medical profession to establish for itself the right to determine healthcare need and to set priorities for health spending through its position as 'gatekeepers' within the new state structures of healthcare provision. Other OECD countries also show a consistent pattern of disproportionate spending on in-patient or 'secondary' care (largely within the setting of a hospital). This pattern reflects the historical dominance and autonomy of the profession within healthcare organisations, and the influence of the biomedical model of disease which focuses solely on the detailed diagnosis and clinical management of sick individuals/patients. The influence of this 'biomedical model' has been one of the main reasons why addressing the social and environmental factors that shape ill-health at a population level has not, until relatively recently, been a priority within most developed countries. The average proportion of spending on public health is just 2.9 percent of total healthcare budgets in OECD countries (OECD, 2005). Ambulatory services in primary care and home-based care (largely neglected in most OECD countries) also receive relatively small proportions of overall healthcare expenditure. This pattern of expenditure, which gives preference

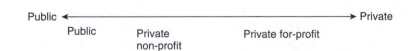

Figure 6.9 Health service providers – range of organisational forms

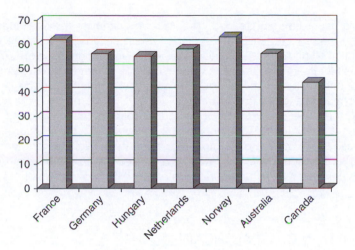

Figure 6.10 In-patient percentage share of healthcare spending 2003 (OECD, 2005)

to in-patient hospital-based secondary care, can be found across virtually all developed countries; this pattern is illustrated in Figure 6.10.

Patient access to services and the availability of choice are factors which reflect the different forms of provision. As discussed above, SHI systems usually offer the choice of doctor or hospital, whilst those countries which have tax funded national health services such as Britain utilise a referral system in which the General Practitioner (GP) in Primary Care acts as a 'gatekeeper' limiting patient choice. Nevertheless, it would be a mistake to see the availability of choice as a function of the organisation of funding of healthcare systems. For example, in the 1990s, the Swedish government expanded the choices that were already available to patients so that they could freely choose both the doctor and institution for medical treatment; although it has a tax-based national health service. A key element of the New Labour government 'modernisation' of the NHS in Britain is also a concern with widening patient choice, whereas the Dutch SHI-funded system has adopted a GP referral system offers only a low level of patient choice (Blank and Burau, 2004: 76).

ACTIVITY

Read the paper by Degos, L. et al. – 'Can France keep its patients happy?' *British Medical Journal* (2008) vol. 336: 254–257). This is paper is free to download at www.bmj.com.

In this paper Laurent Degos and colleagues examine the challenges now faced by the French healthcare system. French continues to get the highest satisfaction ratings of any EU healthcare system, largely because of its freedom of access for users of the service without referral. However, the system is now facing a serious funding crisis as a consequence of maintaining this high level of performance and quality of care.

Read the paper then, based upon your reading of this chapter as well as chapters 4 and 5, identify one aspect of the reforms that have occurred within the British NHS over the past decade that you think might benefit the French system as it is currently constituted, and one element of the French system that you think should be incorporated into the NHS.

REGULATION OF HEALTHCARE SYSTEMS

While the analysis of the finance and service provision dimensions can draw upon quantitative (OECD data) measures of the changes in the role of the state in healthcare, the concept of 'regulation' is much more qualitative in nature. As a conceptual tool, regulation is used in a variety of ways in the health policy literature, but broadly speaking the concept is utilised in order to explain the processes associated with the management of the relationships that exist between the variety of social and organisational actors within a healthcare system. These are relationships that are highly contextual and subject to constant change, and as such cannot be easily quantified. There are a number of regulatory models. In one form, regulation is achieved directly through the imposition of mandatory rules with a strong top-down of command and control role for the state. Regulation can also be achieved through the creation of incentives for competition within a healthcare market, or it can occur through the building of organisational networks that become mutually dependent upon one another (Saltman, 2002).

The history of the development of state regulation begins in the mid- to late nineteenth century when regulatory agencies were created to oversee factory working, public health, fire safety, manufacturing standards and many other areas of industry and commerce. State regulation really expanded after the Second World War when it was extended to consumer rights, environmental protection, anti-discrimination rights, urban planning and many other areas of social life. It has been estimated that by the mid-1990s in Britain there were 135 regulatory agencies overseeing the performance of the public sector, spending between them £770 million a year (representing 0.3 percent of total government expenditure); quadruple the level of public sector regulation that had existed in 1975 (Hood et al., 1999).

There are several explanations found within organisational theory concerning the widespread use of forms of regulation within healthcare systems. Firstly, an external regulatory strategy is one solution for organisations that have a weak or loose managerial hierarchy. Here, regulation may assist the pursuit of corporate objectives (such as raising performance) which might otherwise be met with resistance by staff if pursued by the internal management of a local organisation. Secondly, organisation size can dictate the requirement for regulation. National healthcare systems are large-scale organisations with complex bureaucratic structures, but healthcare is something that is difficult to effectively and efficiently deliver through a conventional hierarchical structure. Regulation can provide an alternative or supplementary mechanism for performance management enabling these large organisations to be managed as a network, chain or set of smaller organisations. From this perspective, the NHS, for example, would be seen not as one organisation but as a network or confederations of about 1000 organisations – trusts, health authorities and so on. Thus, rather than the Department of Health attempting to performance manage the health service through a traditional bureaucratic hierarchy, '… regulatory bodies or agencies are created that take on much of that task of performance management, working to an overall strategy that is set centrally' (Walshe, 2003: 31).

A wide range of forms of organisational regulation can be found across European healthcare systems, reflecting the differing relationships that exist between financing bodies (central government, sickness funds, private insurance companies), service providers (public, not-for-profit agencies, private companies), and service users in these countries. However, at the centre of this regulatory triangle is the medical profession. The demand for healthcare has traditionally been controlled by the clinical decisions of doctors who decide which services should be made available to patients. Over the past two decades, this discretionary power over healthcare resources has been subject to much greater constraint and scrutiny, through the development of new regulatory powers for both national and local healthcare management structures.

In examining the forms of regulation that exist within the German and the UK healthcare systems, for example, a number of significant differences emerge (Rothgang et al., 2005). In terms of healthcare coverage, the establishment of the NHS in the UK brought about universal coverage which has remained the case to the present. In Germany, despite the existence of a SHI system since 1883, many social groups were excluded from the system by virtue of their employment situation. The increase that occurred in public healthcare coverage since the 1970s only came about because the state intervened to regulate the financing bodies. The German state also intervened in the SHI system in the early 1990s to introduce free choice of sickness funds for the insured population with the goal of reducing overall costs. Alternatively, the introduction of the internal market by the Conservative government in the UK can be seen as an attempt to limit the central regulation of service provision and devolving control to local trusts. This is a process that on the surface has continued through the New Labour government 'modernisation' process, although in practice such forms of 'decentralisation' often serve to strengthen regulation from the centre (see Chapter 8 for a detailed discussion of this process). In Germany, the central state has been much more reluctant to intervene to induce the self-regulated corporatist system into becoming more effective in service delivery.

IS THERE A PROCESS OF CONVERGENCE OCCURRING WITHIN EUROPEAN HEALTHCARE SYSTEMS?

A major question confronting comparative health policy analysts is whether it is possible to discern a 'convergence' in the forms and structures of healthcare finance, provision, and regulation present within EU member-states' healthcare systems. This would be convergence towards what has been described by the OECD as the 'public contract' model of health-care organisation and delivery (OECD, 1992). The possible convergence towards such a model is attributed to its functionality, that is its capacity to combine cost containment with efficiency in allocating resources in the face of global economic changes occurring at the end of the twentieth century (Mohan, 1996).

Those supporting the idea of policy convergence point to the role played by process of 'policy learning' and the transfer of ideas ('ideational convergence') across different countries in response to common challenges faced by national healthcare systems (which are identified above). That is, countries with comparable economic, social and political structures such as exist amongst the pre-2004 EU member-states, have much to learn from each other in relation to the impact of organisational change. As Freeman has argued: 'Getting it right in health policy – ensuring universal access to high quality healthcare without breaking the bank – makes for a significant competitive advantage, in the domestic political arena as well as in the international economy' (2000b: 5). Whilst convergence is avowedly a generalised macro-system theory, the concept also points to the role played by institutional agencies working within and across national boundaries in the transfer or 'diffusion' of ideas concerning the management of healthcare systems. The role of the World Bank in shaping health policy in developing countries as part of the terms of providing national loans is well understood, but the role of such supra-governmental organisations in developed countries is a more recent development. The ability of the European Union Commission to intervene in national policy formation is formally limited to the cross-border mobility of goods and services, competitive practices within the single market, and issuing health and safety directives such as that pertaining to working hours. However, in recent years it has also been increasingly active (following the setting-up of the European Observatory on Healthcare Systems) in promoting the diffusion of a set of ideas which seek to frame policy problems and their solutions in particular ways (Blank and Burau, 2004: 212).

Nevertheless, as Freeman has argued, whilst convergence theory may explain why there should be pressure for organisational reform within health systems, it says much less about whether it will occur within particular countries or the form that it will take (2000b: 5). The concept of structural 'path-dependency' (discussed as a key concept in relation to the role of the state in Chapter 2) lends support to this position, in that this theory asserts that any assessment of the processes involved in the development of national healthcare systems has to take into account factors beyond the current internal dynamics of funding and provision. The notions of historical contingency or 'embeddedness' (Wilsford, 1994) also point to the importance of past (nationally specific) policies that become institutionalised within systems and which serve to shape emerging policy responses, building on what is already there.

Certainly convergence towards an EU ideal-type model of healthcare is unlikely to be on the cards in the medium to long-term in Eastern Europe, as EU financial transfers to these countries are much smaller than those that went to Portugal, Ireland and Greece in the 1980s. In the period 2004–06, the 'old' 15 member states contributed an average of only €26 per citizen per year into the EU budget for enlargement. As a consequence, the welfare state provisions for citizens in the majority of these post-2004 Eastern EU member-states, as Timothy Garton Ash (2007: 39) has noted, exists mainly on paper not in reality.

SUMMARY

The purpose of this chapter has been to move beyond studying policy developments within the British NHS in isolation from developments occurring in healthcare systems in countries experiencing similar challenges and demands. Whilst many of the problems and solutions have been similar across EU member-states, it has been argued that the important historical, political and cultural differences that exist between these countries continue to be reflected in the distinct forms that healthcare finance, provision, and regulation take within each country. And, whilst there is evidence that there is some convergence towards a 'public contract' form of healthcare system, the differences that continue to exist between countries demands that a more measured and detailed analysis of policy development in each particular country is undertaken.

FURTHER READING

Blank, R. and Burau, V. (2004) *Comparative Health Policy*. Basingstoke: Palgrave Macmillan.

Freeman, R. (2000a) *The Politics of Health in Europe*. Manchester: Manchester University Press

OECD (2006c) *OECD Health Data: Statistics and Indicators for 30 countries*. Paris: OECD.

Rothgang, H., Cacace, M., Grimmeisen, S. and Wendt, C. (2005) 'The Changing Role of the State in Healthcare Systems', *European Review* 13, Supp. No. 1, 187–212.

PART THREE

ISSUES IN HEALTHCARE PROVISION

7 GOVERNING THE MEDICAL PROFESSION

INTRODUCTION

The popular demand for universal healthcare and welfare services created the basis for the establishment of the post-war welfare state in Britain with the NHS at its centre. However, the optimism that these newly created state health and welfare institutions would now be responsive to the health and social needs of the citizenry was gradually eroded with the ascendancy of the medical profession to positions of power within the NHS.

Doctors were a self-regulated profession, largely unaccountable to the public and its representatives. The profession had already enjoyed a high degree of clinical autonomy in the pre-NHS healthcare structures, reflecting their status within society, but the founding of the NHS established their position as 'gatekeepers'. Doctors were now able to determine health need and allocate state healthcare resources according to their clinical discretionary power; this was a position the profession continued to occupy for the next half-century. One of the defining features of the organisational reforms that have occurred within the NHS over the past two decades has been the attempt made by central government to regain control over healthcare resources, moving it through new forms of regulatory practice overseen by newly empowered service managers. As Michael Moran has argued, there are profound issues surrounding resource allocation and power distribution within all healthcare systems changes; '(C)hanges in the government of the medical profession reflect the outcome of the struggles about these issues. The government of doctors, in other words, is a function of the government of medicine' (Moran, 2004: 27).

NATIONAL HEALTH SERVICE OR NATIONAL MEDICAL SERVICE?: THE HEGEMONY OF THE MEDICAL PROFESSION

Long seen as the 'paradigmatic profession' within sociological analysis, studies, such as that carried out by Mary Ann Elston, have argued that one of the main reasons for the medical profession's pre-eminence lies in the fact that it has and remains, 'a publicly mandated and state-backed monopolistic supplier of a valued service' (1990: 58). This view follows on from Larson's (1977) (Weberian-inspired) account of the process of professionalisation which draws attention to the importance of the connection between the creation and maintenance of monopolistic labour market structures. These structures are seen to provide secure institutional arrangements for maintaining the dominant position of the medical profession, and the demand for the specific forms of knowledge possessed by the profession. Similarly, Johnson's (1982) historical account identifies the state as playing a key role in facilitating the development of the professions in the nineteenth century, arising from the trade-off between the profession providing a service for the state and in return the state extending the professions' influence and increasing their membership. The Medical Act of 1858 established the device of registration for those completing an approved training qualification and conferred the title of 'doctor'. The new institution that was created by the 1858 Act to approve professional registration and to uphold ethical standards was the General Medical Council (GMC). This legislation was, '... both instrumentally and symbolically the sign that state power now stood behind those who controlled the Council' (Moran, 2004: 29). Other health and social care occupations, such as nurses, physiotherapists, medical social workers have attempted to emulate this medical model of professionalism, '(H)owever, lacking the doctor's distinctive combination of a highly-regarded body of expertise and skills with a high degree of cohesion and a tradition of forceful political organisation, they were unable to achieve the same status' (Langan, 1998: 10).

Doctors were effectively able to negotiate a 'compact' with the state at the foundation of the NHS, which Klein (1990) famously described as 'the politics of the double bed', referring to the mutual dependency between the government and the medical profession in the new NHS. The newly created NHS depended upon the medical profession not only for their clinical knowledge and skills to deliver services, but also for their expertise in defining and formulating healthcare policy. The compact gave doctors control over the everyday allocation of resources, while the role of the state was confined to deciding the level of overall state funding allocated to the NHS. However, this state–profession compact directly led to a situation, one that has been commented on by many writers over the half-century history of the NHS, whereby the short-term clinical needs of individual patients became prioritised over the long-term health of the nation. The medical profession thus succeeded in shaping the system in their interests, a process that arguably resulted in the creation of a national medical service rather than a national health service.

This state–profession 'compact' first came under threat during the changing economic circumstances of the mid-1970s, when, as a result of a crisis of profitability in the UK economy and subsequent rising unemployment, state resources began to be squeezed in all directions. By the 1980s, the rising cost of the health service had led the Department of Health to begin the process of seriously assessing the best ways in which to maximise the efficient use of limited state resources. This process led onto a detailed examination of the work of doctors, and proposals to improve their 'efficiency and effectiveness'. Inevitably this focus on managing performance led onto attempts to limit the discretionary power of the profession and the dismantlement of the institutions of medical self-regulation that had existed for a century-and-a-half.

Before moving onto a discussion of the ways in which the power of the medical profession began to be challenged within the healthcare system, it is useful to explore the ways in which this dominance and authority has been analysed within the sociological literature. The purpose being not only to conceptualise what is a fundamental feature of the history and organisation of the NHS, but also to interpret the ways in which the more recent attempts by the state to assert its authority over resources has, and continues to be, challenged by the medical profession.

THE DOMINANCE AND AUTONOMY OF
THE MEDICAL PROFESSION

There is now an extensive sociological literature of the health professions reflecting very different points of social theoretical departure.
One approach draws upon a Foucauldian conceptualisation in which
power is essentially relational rather than being an attribute possessed
by individual doctors or the medical profession as a whole. From this
perspective the power of the profession is seen to derive from the dominance
of a biomedical discourse, which shapes the way in which individuals
interpret and respond to their health and illness. Although this relational
understanding of power has been influential, the sociology of the professions
has for a long period been dominated by those working within the
Weberian tradition. This perspective utilises the notions of 'autonomy'
and 'dominance' in order to focus upon the ways in which professions
establish power through the development and maintenance of occupational
boundaries.

It was Eliot Friedson's influential work, '*The Profession of Medicine*'
(1970), that firmly established what was to became known as the
'professional dominance' or 'power approach' model. This approach,
strongly influenced by Weberian notions of power, knowledge, and status,
consciously sought to challenge the then prevailing conceptualisations of
the medical profession. Up to this time, the two dominant perspectives of
professions were the Parsonian functionalist view of an ethical profession
using its expert knowledge rationally and altruistically within a rule-
bound organic society, and the Durkheimian professional 'traits' model.
Friedson was concerned primarily with the day-to-day world of the medical
profession which, whilst employing abstract professional principles at the
discursive level of professional training, was in practice actively engaged
in the process of maintaining and developing its power and autonomy.
This approach was to become the orthodoxy in sociological analyses of
the professions (MacDonald, 1995: 5). Friedson argued that the power
of medicine in modern societies did not derive from a social consensus
around its gate-keeping role in legitimating sickness but rested upon two
essentially self-serving pillars. The first being its 'autonomy', or the ability
of the profession to control its own work activities. The second relates to the
control the profession exercises over the work activities of other healthcare
occupations within the division of labour of healthcare systems, namely its
'dominance'.

This model of professional dominance was subject to an increasing
criticism in the 1980s as sociologists attempted to describe and explain
the apparent decline in the autonomy of the professions as a whole.

Two models in particular achieved some prominence. First, what was termed the 'proletarianisation' thesis, which was associated with the work of McKinlay and Arches (1985). This model, identified two key changes as being responsible for the medical profession's perceived loss of dominance within the healthcare system: (1) the then recent development of 'managerialism' within healthcare systems, which was seen to have reduced doctor's control over clinical decision-making and (2) the process of de-skilling in the face of increased specialisation and technological developments within the medical field. Together, these processes were seen as technicising the role of doctors such they were becoming simply one group of employees (albeit one with a high degree of expertise) within the healthcare system. The second model of professional decline was termed the 'deprofessionalisation' model and was associated with the work of Haug and Lavin (1983). These authors argued that the knowledge gap between doctors and patients had narrowed, and that consequently there had been a shift in power towards the healthcare consumer. Haug and Lavin argued that this general trend was leading to a diminishing of the cultural authority and health knowledge monopoly of medicine. Both these models of professional decline were developed as specific commentaries on the situation of US medicine. However, this does not necessarily rule out their applicability to the state system of healthcare in Britain, especially following the introduction of the internal market in the NHS in 1990, and they are still reproduced in the sociological literature assessing the medical professions.

More recent work is hesitant about drawing general assumptions about any long-term loss of power by the medical profession. Elston's (1991) work developed Friedson's (1970) previous limited notion of professional autonomy. She identifies three distinct categories of autonomy: 'economic autonomy' as the ability to determine remuneration, 'political autonomy' as the ability to influence policy choices, and 'clinical autonomy' as the profession's right to set its own standards and to control clinical performance. Elston was then able to argue that a decline in one of the forms of medical autonomy does not necessarily effect change in other areas of autonomy and status. Elston maintained that whilst the 1990 internal market reforms within the NHS (described in Chapter 4 above) challenged the post-war political consensus over the organisation of the NHS and the unregulated role of the medical profession and, as such, represented a decline in the political autonomy of medicine, but not, however, its continuing clinical control over health resources.

Friedson (1994, 2001) has shifted his analytical position concerning the relative power of the medical profession over the years following the publication of *The Profession of Medicine* in 1970. He has more recently argued that this dominance is best understood by an assessment of the actual work of doctors within the context of the healthcare division of labour. Friedson's (1994) concern is thus with the microlevel of power, and here he identifies what he terms a 'zone of discretion' specific to medical work. At this level, a professional monopoly over certain skills ensures that even rank-and-file doctors are able to maintain a large amount of discretion in their daily work vis-à-vis other health workers. Together, these discretionary powers usually enable doctors to prevent encroachment upon their clinical autonomy, whether that comes from managerialist attempts to monitor their performance or from the nursing or midwifery professions in taking on aspects of work that doctors regard as being within their prerogative.

Friedson further argues that, if the profession is seen in terms of being a 'corporate body', rather than primarily in terms of the work practices of individual practitioners, then its power has not been seriously undermined over the last two decades of organisational change. Nevertheless, he does recognise that the divisions within the profession have increased, not merely between rival specialisms but between the elite and the rank-and-file. This process of 'internal stratification' is seen as an adaptive response to external pressures from state and market to limit the spiralling costs of medical diagnosis and treatment. While the profession has maintained its autonomy at the 'corporate' level of the healthcare system, the price for this control has been the opening-up of internal policing systems in order to monitor standards of individual performance of the profession. In Britain, evidence of these developments also came with the Conservative government's 1990 NHS reforms, which, whilst giving the new groups of professional managers a greater role in decision-making, also effectively endorsed the medical profession's control over its own standards and activities of work. Although a new process of clinical audit was introduced, the medical profession was allowed to manage this process internally. In addition, many senior doctors were incorporated into formal management roles, given titles such as 'clinical director', and charged with formally managing the work of other doctors and healthcare professionals.

Finally, whilst acknowledging the force of Friedson's argument concerning the adaptability of the senior members of the medical profession in the face of the managerialist reforms to the organisation of healthcare, a point must be reached when it is possible to say that 'things ain't what they used to be'. In relation to the traditional dominance and autonomy enjoyed by doctors within the NHS, that point has now clearly been reached with the introduction by the New Labour government of national standards and frameworks of treatment and care, as well as the imminent imposition of a reform of medicine's self-regulatory bodies.

NEW CHALLENGES TO THE DOMINANCE OF THE MEDICAL PROFESSION

The challenges to the continuing dominance of the medical profession within healthcare systems come from a range of sources. First is the impact upon the clinical autonomy of the profession due to the introduction of new regulatory mechanisms designed to rationalise and more closely manage healthcare provision. This has had important consequences in terms of a changing balance of authority within healthcare; here termed 'governance' (outlined as a Key Concept below). Secondly, in terms of a loss of public trust and confidence in the profession following a number of high profile medical scandals. Thirdly, the impact of greater demands for patient involvement in their own care reflecting an end to the traditional deference offered to the profession, and frustration with the limited communication concerning treatment. Finally, the consequences of a changing division of labour arising out of various technical and rationalisation processes occurring with healthcare systems.

KEY CONCEPT: GOVERNANCE

In the policy literature the constructs of governance and regulation are sometimes deployed to describe what outwardly would appear to be similar sets of processes; this can cause some confusion for the unwary. In the context of this textbook, 'regulation' is utilised to describe the *exercise of authority* by state agencies through the establishment of rules which serve to control and/or incentivise the activities of both social and organisational actors within the state healthcare system. 'Governance' on the other hand, is an analytical construct that is utilised here to describe the processes associated with the *relationship of authority* existing between the State, the public/health service users, and the health and welfare professions entrusted with the implementation of policies that impact upon the lives of these citizens.

At its simplest level then, governance describes the way in which organisations and the people working in them *relate* to each other. Although a more complex definition would also draw attention to '(t)he arrangements by which authority and function are allocated, and rights and obligations established and regulated and through which policies and practices are effected' (Gray, 2004: 6). Different modes or types of governance can also be identified. These can include a control and command 'mode' of governance

(Continued)

(*Continued*)

which is very typical of traditional forms of top-down government or organisational bureaucracy. Secondly, a mode of governance which focuses on building a shared value system or frame of reference within an organisation or service, which some might describe as 'soft' governance. Thirdly, a contractual mode based upon an inducement–contribution exchange between different parties, typically found in market-led services.

Within the NHS, issues of governance are reflected in the way in which the interests and 'social rights of participation' of the various 'actors' in healthcare are balanced one against the other. The role of the state being to resolve the tensions existing between the traditional forms of clinical decision-making autonomy exercised by medical professionals, and the demands for greater public control over their activities; albeit that the state is not a neutral player in this process of governance. New forms of healthcare governance are also reflected in the changing nature of the relationship existing between the individual responsibility of the citizen-users of health services, and the formal responsibilities of the welfare state towards its citizens. Understanding these processes also requires that we look at the 'intersections and tensions' between the users/citizens, health professions, and the state (Kuhlmann, 2006: 8).

PROFESSIONAL REGULATION

In Chapter 6, modes of regulation were identified as one dimension (the others being finance and provision) of an analytical framework that could be deployed to comparatively assess European healthcare systems on the basis of their core or functional processes. Regulation in the context of state healthcare systems was defined as an external approach to management or control of performance improvement (relating to both organisational and individual behaviours) from outside the healthcare delivery organisation itself through processes of inspection.

Across all levels of healthcare activity, the NHS was largely free of any form of regulatory intrusion until the late 1980s, the organisation being directly accountable through a traditional bureaucratic hierarchy to central government. The noticeable exceptions to this lack of formal regulation over healthcare delivery were the Health Advisory Service (HAS) and the Audit Commission. The HAS was created in 1969 in response to a series of scandals involving the ill-treatment of patients in long-stay institutions, and was given the responsibility for inspecting services to the mentally ill, the elderly and those with learning disabilities. The Audit Commission and National Audit Office were created in the 1980s, their regulatory objective was to ensure public money was spent as Parliament intended, as well as improving financial control within public service organisations.

The use of regulatory instruments to specifically control the activities of the medical profession is a relatively recent development within the NHS. The state having established and given the GMC statutory powers in 1858 as the medical profession's self-regulatory body, withdrew from any further regulation of the profession for more than a century. However, with the economic recession of the mid-1970s, governments of both main political parties began to rethink their open-ended commitment to the pursuance of a universal health and social welfare system. Yet, it was not until its third term in office that the Conservative government published the White Paper, *Working for Patients* (DoH, 1989), with its proposals for the creation of an internal market in healthcare. As described in Chapter 4, the BMA reaction to these proposals was immediate and vociferous, and a well-funded campaign of opposition was launched. Nevertheless, in practice whilst the organisational restructuring resulted in a greater role for the new professional managers in decision-making concerning the use of healthcare resources, the medical profession's control over its own standards and activities of work was not fundamentally challenged. Indeed, arguably the GP fundholding schemes endorsed this aspect of self-regulation, despite the introduction of mandatory medical audit.

The New Labour government did not set out to overtly regulate the work of doctors on coming into power in 1997, but it did introduce a new professional accountability and quality assurance structure known as the 'clinical governance framework'. A key pillar of this framework was the promotion of an 'evidence-based practice'. The medical profession had acknowledged the necessity of moving away from traditional forms of routinised practices which often lead to unsafe and ineffective patient interventions, yet integrating best evidence into practice has not always been straightforward. There are important barriers to doctors delivering evidence-based care, not least of which are the demands associated with keeping abreast of an ever-widening literature. The clinical governance framework was also constructed with the aim of encouraging doctors to think in wider strategic terms about the efficient use of healthcare resources. The prevailing view being that the medical profession had historically only ever been able to conceive of clinical need at the level of the individual patient.

Under the rubric of 'modernisation', the New Labour government has, since 1998, developed not just a clinical governance framework, but also other forms of regulation which have enabled local and national managers to more closely control the discretionary power of the medical profession (Crinson, 2004: 43). In 1999, the National Institute for Clinical Excellence (NICE) was created and charged by the Department of Health with appraising a particular drug or 'medical technology' where its use may have a 'significant impact on NHS resources', or where 'there is confusion or uncertainty over its value' (DoH, 1998b). This development has subsequently brought about a significant diminution of the ability of doctors to prescribe medicines they determine are the most clinically effective on grounds of cost (the role of NICE is discussed in detail in Chapter 8). The introduction of a whole set of National Service Frameworks (NSFs) for different medical conditions has also played an important role in regulating clinical work through the setting of incentivised clinical guidelines.

ACTIVITY

One of the key principles associated with the practice of 'New Managerialism' in the NHS, is that all occupational groups must subsume their own professional interests in order to meet the objectives and goals of the organisation as a whole.

Following your reading of the preceding sections of this chapter, try and identify three features associated with medical professional autonomy that are potential points of conflict with this managerial approach.

PUBLIC TRUST AND PATIENT SAFETY

Public trust in the medical profession has undoubtedly been severely diminished following the outcome of the public inquiries into the Shipman Murders (Shipman, 2004), and children's heart surgery at Bristol Royal Infirmary (Kennedy, 2001). The Kennedy Inquiry pointed to the ways in which the dominance of senior doctors within an institution can lead to a 'club culture' and an imbalance of power between medical and other members of staff. This was recognised as contributing to a lack of teamworking and the failure to work together in the best interests of the patient.

Consequently in 2007 the government published its White Paper, which set out its programme of reform to the system for the regulation of health professionals, with its primary concern being to ensure patient safety and quality of care (DoH, 2007a). Many of the reform proposals will require primary legislation, including the restructuring of the GMC, and new licensing arrangements for doctors. It has been made quite clear to the medical profession that if it is to retain any measure of control over its clinical activities, there will be no going back to the behind-closed-doors self-regulatory system that it was able to maintain throughout the years of Conservative government rule.

CHANGING HEALTHCARE GOVERNANCE – THE CHALLENGE OF PATIENT-CENTRED MEDICINE

One of the major emergent challenges to the hegemony of the medical profession within the NHS has been the raising of public expectations about the service they receive, and a greater willingness to question the profession's right to determine health need. It is difficult to be sociologically precise about the reasons why this process should have occurred over the last two decades, but certainly both the New Labour governments since 1997, and the previous Conservative government, played their part in encouraging greater public and patient involvement, albeit for their own political purposes. At an ideological level, although not at a practical level, both Labour and Conservative governments have promoted the rights of the patient citing this as one of the primary factors in their health service reform programmes. The first example of this process in more recent times was the 'Patients Charter' introduced by the John Major Conservative government in 1992, a copy of which was sent to every household in the country setting out service standards, expectations and patient rights.

As the traditional paternalistic model of clinical decision-making came be seen as outdated as a consequence of shifts in the relationship of healthcare governance towards a greater role for the patient, so the patient–doctor consultation began to be reformulated in terms of the new 'patient-centred' strategies. The principles of patient-centred medicine, are now a core element in the curriculum taught to new medical students, and there is evidence that it is has been incorporated into clinical practice in primary care (noting the conclusions of the case study set out in Chapter 3, which pointed to these principles coming into conflict with incentivised clinical treatment guidelines for GPs). This approach stresses the importance of doctors understanding patients' experiences of their illness as well as any other relevant social and psychological factors. What is known as the 'shared decision-making' model shares a number of similarities with patient-centred medicine. However, the concept also includes patients' active involvement in the treatment decision. The 'shared decision-making' model has four main characteristics as follows: both the patient and the doctor are involved; both parties share information; both parties take steps to build a consensus about the preferred treatment; an agreement is reached on the treatment to implement.

However, a study of doctor–patient communication about medication (Stevenson et al., 2000) which looked specifically at the first two of the four characteristics of the model (participation in the consultation in terms of sharing information about, and views of medicines), found little evidence that doctors and patients participate in the consultation in this way. GPs' perceptions of both their (dominant) role and the behaviour of patients (deferring to doctors' advice) were found to reduce the likelihood of shared decision-making. The explanation offered by GPs who participated in the study as to why they had not engaged in shared decision-making included lack of time and other organisational pressures in general practice. It was also suggested that patients expect their problems to be solved, and that the solution should include a prescription. Thus, there is a belief that patients lack the will or ability to participate in treatment decision-making (a position which is well documented in the medical sociology literature). The study concluded there was no basis upon which to build a consensus about the preferred treatment and reach an agreement on which treatment to implement. More recent research concurs with these findings. A study by Rogers et al. (2005) of patients self-managing their chronic condition and their relative satisfaction with the support received from their doctor suggested that a number of factors served to inhibit effective patient-centred consultations. These included the failure of doctors to fully incorporate the expressed need relevant to people's self-management activities, and an interpretation of patient self-management as constituting compliance with medical instructions. One of the important contributions of these sociological papers is the finding that professional culture still plays an important role in perpetuating certain core beliefs, for example the idea that the doctor knows what is in the best interests of the patient, which act to hinder the development of a truly patient-centred healthcare service (Crinson, 2008).

CHANGING PROFESSIONAL BOUNDARIES

The 'modernisation' programme for the NHS was predicated on the assumption that the goal of greater resource efficiency and wider choice for patients could not be achieved with the existing health workforce structure and traditional forms of professional practice. Derek Wanless's report on the future of the health service, which was commissioned by the Treasury in 2000, concluded that:

> The number and mix of staff in the health service is a major determinant of the volume and quality of care ... a health service without the right number of people, with the right skills, in the right locations will not deliver a high quality, comprehensive service to patients over the next two decades. (Wanless, 2001)

Celia Davies has asserted that the changes that have subsequently begun to be introduced in the working practices of the healthcare professions represent the most fundamental development that has occurred in its sixty year history:

> For many people working inside the NHS, the 1980s and early 1990s felt like a period of total revolution in healthcare. New vocabularies of business management pervaded thinking. Markets and managerialism came to the fore, and competition and contracting were the order of the day. Yet, despite the new words and employment relations, the division of labour in delivering patient care remained much the same ... the real revolution came after 1997, when New Labour began not just to reshape once again the overall organisational arrangements of healthcare, but to redesign the workforce. Assumptions about the professional autonomy of doctors, about the hierarchies and divisions of labour between and among other health professions that had survived successive health service reorganisations of earlier decades began to be cast aside. The workforce of the future seemed set to look remarkably different from the workforce of the present (Davies, 2003: 1)

Modernisation of the structures and organisation of the NHS was seen to necessitate a new approach to utilisation of local health resources (including market forces), and a greater openness towards inter-agency and inter-professional collaboration. From these working assumptions emerged the government's '*Agenda for Change*' policy for the NHS workforce (DoH, 2004b) which sought to develop a new pay and incentive system that would provide more flexibility for the NHS employers, giving them the ability to:

- Design jobs around the needs of patients rather than around grading definitions;
- Define the core skills and knowledge they want staff to develop in each job;
- Pay extra when they face recruitment and retention difficulties.

Here the concept of 'boundary-setting' has a particular relevance to an understanding of those inter-disciplinary interactions that have traditionally marked the healthcare division of labour. The traditional distinction between medicine and nursing was said to be between treatment and care, but this boundary is seen to have become an indistinct one as nurses have increasingly been encouraged by the Department of Health to take on aspects of doctors' work, especially within primary care.

There is also now a much stronger emphasis being placed by the Department of Health on inter-professionalism and collaborative practice. This shift in approach was set out in the guidance document, *A Health Service of All the Talents: Developing the NHS Workforce: a Framework for Lifelong Learning for the NHS* (DoH, 2000a). The current skill mix of healthcare staff is now seen to be unable to meet the ever-increasing and new demands being placed on the healthcare system. Recent shifts in Department of Health workforce planning seek to focus on integrated inter-professional or inter-agency working rather than on traditional medical profession-centred planning. These shifts in planning are being conducted alongside a critical reappraisal of the types of roles and expertise needed for the healthcare workforce of the future. What are termed 'Care Group Workforce Teams' (CGWT) have now been set up by the Department of Health in order to identify national staffing issues affecting particular services and develop plans on how they ought to be addressed. Recommendations have now been produced by the Department of Health on the skills and competencies required to deliver on all the NSF guidelines in the areas of cancer, maternity and gynaecology services, heart disease, long-term conditions including diabetes, mental health, and services for older people. Complimentary to this process, the Department of Health (2000a) has for some time been encouraging the development of shared learning in the education and training of new health and social care professionals (including medical students). Following the recommendation of Wanless's Final Report (2002), nurses are now increasingly being encouraged by the Department of Health to take on aspects of doctors' work especially within primary care ('enhanced roles'). These developments clearly represent a significant challenge to the traditional hegemony of the medical profession within healthcare teams.

SUMMARY

This chapter has sought to focus attention on the ways in which the traditional hegemony of the medical profession over resources and healthcare needs planning and implementation has been increasingly challenged by both Conservative and New Labour governments. The primary driver of these developments is the necessity for the state to ensure greater control over health resources and efficiency in their use in the face of rising demands and raised public expectations about the quality of healthcare delivery. The modernisation developments outlined in this chapter are undoubtedly leading to a reconfiguration of the NHS workforce that will have a fundamental impact on the role of the healthcare professional of the future.

FURTHER READING

Friedson, E. (2001) *Professionalism: The Third Logic*. Cambridge: Policy Press.
Gray, A. and Harrison, S. (eds) (2004) *Governing Medicine: Theory and Practice*. Maidenhead: Open University Press.

Kennedy, I. (2001) *The Report of the Bristol Royal Infirmary Inquiry*. London: The Stationery Office. Available at: http://www.bristol-inquiry.org.uk/final_report/rpt_print.htm

Stevenson, F., Barry, C., Britten, N., Barber, N. and Bradley, C. (2000) 'Doctor-patient communication about drugs: the evidence for shared decision making', *Social Science and Medicine* 50: 829–840.

8 MANAGING THE PERFORMANCE OF THE NHS

BACKGROUND: SYSTEM REFORM AND ORGANISATIONAL PERFORMANCE

The NHS in the mid-1990s was increasingly seen as failing to meet the raised public expectations of a modern healthcare system: this was tangibly represented by the ever-growing waiting lists for treatment. This general disillusionment was also keenly felt by health service staff, whose trade unions and professional associations strongly and publicly asserted the argument that the workforce were not being provided with the resources to address these rising demands for healthcare – a shortfall that was made ever more acute because of the ever-spiralling costs of new medical technology and medicines. This process of 'under-funding' was seen as overriding any impact that the organisational reforms (the 'internal market') of the NHS introduced in 1990 by the Conservative government may have had in providing incentives for efficiency in the use of resources. The New Labour government was returned to power in 1997 in large part because of its electoral commitment to restore funding and confidence in the NHS.

This commitment to moving away from the cycle of under-funding was given a concrete form with the publication of *The NHS Plan* (DoH, 2000b), which set out a timetable for achieving healthcare funding levels comparable to other European Union states. However, it was made clear in *The NHS Plan* that this significant increase in state funding was given on the basis that the 'modernisation' process set out in the ten-year plan would be fully implemented. Central to this process was the development of a performance management system designed to both regulate and provide incentives for efficiency and productivity amongst local service providers. The model of performance management has emerged in a rather piecemeal way since the publication of *The NHS Plan* in 2000, could be said to be characterised by forms of what is termed 'arm's length regulation' (for example the work of NICE and the Healthcare Commission) as well as the setting of targets and guidelines by the centre. This form of organisational governance enabled the Department of Health to scrutinise and shape the organisational behaviour of the NHS, yet left the day-to-day responsibility for corrective action to improve performance with the organisation itself (Hood et al., 1999; Hood and Scott, 2000). Thus, in principle this 'arm's length' or 'once-removed regulatory state' (as it has been termed) avoids the political problems that were experienced by the previous Conservative government, who retained ministerial responsibility for local failures in healthcare provision following the introduction of the 'internal market.' However, there is also evidence (presented below) that points also to the emergence of new 'dysfunctionalities' within local organisations following the introduction of this model of regulation (Bevan, 2006).

A crucial component of this new performance management system is an effective local organisational bureaucratic structure with the authority and power to plan and meet local health needs. This is not, at least in principle, a bureaucracy that conforms to Weber's classic typology of a rule-bound and rigid bureaucratic hierarchy (discussed in Chapter 3). Rather, it is a form of 'managerialism' in which local health service management is given the power and authority (and accountability) that is more characteristic of managers in private sector organisations, in order to achieve the overall objectives of government. The key concept of 'managerialism' is outlined below, as a prelude to discussing the rolling out within the NHS of what has been termed the 'Performance Assessment Framework'.

KEY CONCEPT – MANAGERIALISM

'Managerialism' is a method of organisational administration that was widely adopted across European states in the 1980s and 1990s in order to reform public sector organisations. The process of managerialism was seen to be a universal solution to what were perceived to be common problems of inefficiency, incompetence and chaos characteristic of the public provision of public health and welfare services.

Managerialism as an ideal-type administrative ideology or doctrine, is typically associated with a set of practices which promote a hands-on or business-like style of management in which decision-making power becomes the prerogative of managers: '... discretion' as attached to a managerial rather than professional calculus' (Clarke, 1998: 176). The doctrine of managerialism emphasises the importance of having explicit output controls (to be measured by explicit performance indices), decentralisation of decision-making, and the extolling of virtues of competition between these disaggregated units. There is also typically a commitment to the creation of a 'transparent' organisation in which all employees are expected to strive to meet the 'corporate' objectives; loyalty of staff is primarily to the organisation itself rather than to some more esoteric notion of public service 'ethic'. Within policy analysis, this set of practices is termed the 'new public management' (NPM), and its use as a concept within the UK is usually credited to the work of Hood (1991).

Clarke (1998; 2004) has argued that the introduction of managerialism into the public healthcare sector represented more than the imposition of rationalist business methods, its introduction was primarily about refashioning the role of the state in the delivery of healthcare. The NPM should therefore not be seen as another step in some evolutionary development of public service organisations, nor as simply just one component of a neoliberal politically driven reform of the health and welfare, but rather as a 'distinct formation' with its own dynamic. In this analysis, managerialism is presented as the 'cement' that can hold together and coordinate the increasingly 'dispersed form' of the state in which a wide range of agents and organisations are now involved in the provision of services. The process of state reform associated with new forms of governance, decentralisation and devolution, contractualisation and competition between providers, is seen to require the employment of new systems of control at a distance. In this process, the management of 'performance' has become framed as one of the most important ways of achieving organisational control, through new forms of scrutiny, inspection and audit (Clarke, 2004: 129).

However, as the NPM enters its 'middle age' analysts are beginning to digest the burgeoning literature on the practice of managerialism in the public sector. A paper by Hood and Peters (2004) has identified a number of what

(Continued)

(*Continued*)

they term 'paradoxes', 'surprises', and contradictions associated with the operation of this system of public sector management. The first 'paradox' is associated with the focus on controls over organisational 'outputs' through the use of performance indicators. Unintended effects result from the fact that public service activities such as healthcare are not readily observable and cannot be treated as a pure process of 'production'. Imposing a uniform set of controls is seen to result in an over-similarity and conformity between organisations, which is the opposite of the radical innovation and competitiveness that NPM was designed to promote within the public sector. The second 'paradox' concerns the original promotion of the NPM as a method of depoliticising public management by positioning central government control at 'arms-length' through the transferring of direct responsibility for public service delivery to managers. Paradoxically this increasingly led to politicians intervening in the appointment (and sacking) of managers in order to retain control over policy implementation processes (this process has been very apparent within the NHS in recent years). The third 'paradox' relates to the claim that NPM was 'results orientated' as opposed to the rule-based and 'process-driven' routines of traditional bureaucratic management. The conclusions of a cross-national study (Pollitt et al., 1999) is cited to demonstrate that in many cases the procedural rules on public management have actually been augmented through greater regulation; a basic case of 'goal displacement.' Hood and Peters (2004: 275) go on to suggest that the paradoxes described above could be accounted for at least in part by March and Olsen's (1976) famous 'garbage can model' of organisational non-linearity (outlined in Chapter 3 above). This model asserts that the mixture of complex systems with vague middle-level goals, combined with the culture clashes of a fluid cast of participating players, inevitably produce unpredictable results and shifting agendas.

CONSTRUCTING A PERFORMANCE ASSESSMENT AND MANAGEMENT FRAMEWORK IN THE NHS

Performance management as a strategic construct first came to prominence in relation to the delivery of public services in Britain in the mid-1980s. In the context of the NHS, the report of the Griffiths Inquiry (DHSS, 1983) into the management of the NHS (outlined in Chapter 4) concluded that although the health service lacked effective control systems this problem could be remedied by clarifying the management hierarchy and creating general managers who could integrate clinical and financial knowledge. While the Conservative government swiftly implemented the Inquiry's recommendations concerning the introduction of general managers across the service, it took a little longer to roll out Griffith's other major recommendation, the development of a system of resource management. The 'resource management initiative' (RMI) emerged in 1986, and involved the development of information systems that could provide details of clinical procedure costs and clinician activity in order to support the more effective use (or as many defined it at the time, 'rationing') of resources. However, at the time the information necessary for such a system to function was largely unavailable to managers as it remained locked up within the clinical decision-making autonomy enjoyed by the medical profession. Nevertheless, Griffiths did ultimately have some success in enrolling the participation of the profession in the new form of managerialism. His case was that the general manager posts would provide new career opportunities for doctors and enable them to use their clinical knowledge to shape financial priorities, whereas staying on the outside would mean allowing accountants to impose their financial priorities on clinicians (Dowswell, Harrison and Wright, 2002).

The implementation of many of the management reforms directly recommended by Griffiths is generally judged to have been a policy failure in that it did not achieve the short- to medium-term control over health spending that it was designed to obtain. The reforms did nevertheless establish new principles of clinical and financial management, which laid the ground for future performance reform (Webster, 2002). The first steps in this reform process came about with the introduction by the Conservative government of the *Working for Patients* (DoH, 1989a) 'internal market' reforms which established a new division between 'purchasers' and 'providers' of healthcare. The establishment of this 'internal market' relied in large part upon extending the RMI so that clinical work could become more closely subject to scrutiny through clinical audit and performance monitoring; thus widening the managerial restructuring of the NHS (the question of whether issues of raising quality of care were given the same status as cost-efficiency is explored in detail in Chapter 9). However, although the new purchaser–provider divide was designed to conform to classic economic models of contracting, the internal market was never a truly competitive one. The goal of improving efficiency came to rely upon a process of negotiation between both parties (mainly fundholding GPs and hospital trusts) rather than on the threat of switching to new contractors (Le Grand, Mays and Dixon, 1998).

During the last years of the Conservative government the use of terminology such as 'markets' and 'purchasing' began to be replaced in favour of the concept of 'commissioning' services. This was a shift of emphasis that was to undergo significant development under the New Labour government (a process explored in Chapter 9). In retrospect, the claims that were made at the time concerning the extent to which these reforms improved organisational efficiency appear to have been overplayed.

The 'modernisation' of the NHS instigated by the New Labour government saw the construction, albeit in a piecemeal fashion, of a performance management system which broadened the use of performance indicators in order to meet the government's commitment to raising the quality of, and access to, healthcare. The White Paper, *The New NHS: Modern, Dependable* (DoH, 1997a), published very early in the life of the government, set out the basic principles of health system performance, moving it beyond the concerns of the previous government with adhering to strict budgets, maximisation of patient throughput and reducing waiting times for surgery, to the raising of patient satisfaction and improving clinical quality standards. For the first time in the history of the NHS national performance standards were introduced, and their implementation monitored. Subsequently, a series of explicit targets and instruments were set out in the detailed *NHS Plan* (DoH, 2006). Two new 'arm's length' regulatory agencies were constructed in order to monitor performance and raise clinical standards, the Commission for Health Improvement (CHI) whose remit was to inspect and produce a public report on clinical standards in NHS healthcare organisations, and the National Institute of Clinical Excellence (NICE) whose remit was to produce guidance to clinicians on the clinical and cost effectiveness of medical technologies (a term which covers pharmaceuticals as well diagnostic and therapeutic equipment). In addition, the development of new National Service Frameworks (NSFs) was initiated; these were to be national guidelines for the treatment and management of a range of medical conditions (coronary heart disease, cancer, etc.) and of population groups (e.g., the elderly, children).

Following the publication of *The NHS Plan*, local health service managers were now expected to meet new clinical standards and performance guidelines within the strict financial limits initially set by the Department of Health (note: the New Labour government did not move outside the financial targets set by the previous Conservative government for the first two years of its administration). The newly established Performance Assessment Framework (PAF) was designed to assess the performance of local healthcare organisations in six key areas; health improvement; fair access to services; effective and appropriate delivery of healthcare; health outcomes of NHS care; efficient use of resources; and high quality patient and care-giver experiences. Each key area was given its own set of quantitative indicators and it was announced that annual tables were to be published by the NHS on how each local trust had performed against these measures. This fulfilled the New Labour government commitment to providing the public with easily understandable information on the performance of their local health services. A national fund was established in order to enable NHS trusts to build local capacity towards meeting the new NHS performance targets. This process was intended to initiate a system of 'earned autonomy' for local trusts that was dependent upon their success in meeting the national outcome measures.

Initially local performance was classified on a traffic-light scale of 'green,' 'yellow' or 'red,' with 'green light' organisations being rewarded with greater autonomy. A year later in 2001, this scale was replaced by the system of 'star-ratings' (from zero to three stars). The first annual performance rating for NHS Trusts in England was published by the Department of Health in September 2001 (DoH, 2001b), with the fifth and final set published in 2005 (Healthcare Commission, 2005). Here it should be noted that the responsibility for publishing performance data, including star ratings, was handed to the formally independent body the CHI in 2003, and following its abolition responsibility passed on to the Healthcare Commission. The government abandoned star-ratings for local healthcare organisation performance at the end of 2005, but local performance targets remain and continue to be annually monitored by the Healthcare Commission.

The goal of developing transparent public reporting systems that seek to hold the performance of healthcare providers to account can be found across healthcare systems. However, it has been argued that these approaches;

(a)re premised on the assumption that the provision of comparative quantitative data will deliver genuine improvements, even though there is an absence of hard evidence on the benefits and risks of public disclosure and little in-depth understanding of how these data are perceived, received and acted upon in provider organisations (Mannion, Davies and Marshall, 2005: 18).

Bevan and Hood (2006) have similarly concluded that the policy of organisational regulation by performance target-setting has assumed that priorities can be targeted, and that the part that is measured can stand for the whole, and what is omitted does not matter. Yet,

... typically for defined priorities there will be a few good measures (such as waiting times); a larger group of imperfect measures (such as mortality), the use of which is liable to generate false positive and false negative results; and an even larger group for which no useable data (which applies to the clinical quality of much of healthcare) (Bevan and Hood, 2006: 420).

The evidence for the successful integration of PAF within the day-to-day organisation of local health services is explored below in the section on organisational culture. However, before discussing these local responses an outline of the second element of the modernisation strategy designed to improve the performance and effectiveness of the NHS, the role of 'arm's length' regulatory agencies will be explored.

THE DEVELOPING ROLE OF REGULATORY AGENCIES WITHIN THE MODERNISED NHS: THE WORK OF NICE AND THE HEALTHCARE COMMISSION

The role and remit of the new 'arm's length' agencies and the national system of performance and clinical guidelines measures (to be developed through the National Service Frameworks) was established following the publication of both *The New NHS: Modern, Dependable* (DoH, 1997a) and *The NHS Plan* (DoH, 2000b). In this section we will look at how this new system of regulatory control has developed and performed in relation to healthcare provision since 1997, focusing on the work of the National Institute of Clinical Excellence (NICE) and the Healthcare Commission (formally CHI).

New Labour's White Paper on health service reform, *The New NHS: Modern, Dependable* (DoH, 1997a) proposed the creation of an appraisal body (what was to become NICE) to give 'guidance' to the NHS in appraising new and existing clinical interventions, giving best practice advice and developing clinical audit methodologies. The final details of this role for were then set out in the policy paper, *A First Class Service* (DoH, 1998b), which determined that NICE was to be formally constituted as a Special Health Authority and therefore directly accountable to the Secretary of State for Health. Although a cost-effectiveness approach to health resource allocation decisions had been utilised within the NHS since the 1980s, the implementation of this principle had been less than consistent: with the establishment of NICE this approach was now put on a more systematic footing.

NICE guidance was to be developed utilising the expertise of all stakeholders (NHS management, healthcare professionals, the pharmaceutical and medical technology industry, academics, as well as patients and their carers) and base its recommendations on the best available evidence using a transparent decision-making process. The detailed process of appraising clinical treatments was to involve the commissioning of a review of the published clinical evidence in combination with formal submissions from the stakeholder groups. Consistent with this role, the NICE Appraisal Committees were given the responsibility of appraising both the clinical effectiveness of a particular medical technology as well as its cost effectiveness. To this end, a specially designed economic model was to be employed which estimated the effectiveness of the treatment in terms of the mean cost per quality-adjusted life year (QALY).[1]

A CASE STUDY OF THE WORK OF NICE – BETA INTERFERON AS A TREATMENT FOR MULTIPLE SCLEROSIS

This case study focuses upon the introduction of the use of beta interferon as a drug treatment designed to reduce the inflammatory processes characteristic of MS that occur in the brain and spinal cord. Multiple Sclerosis (MS) is a disabling degenerative neurological disease that affects some 63,000 people in England and Wales, and over 85,000 in the UK as a whole. It can take several forms, but some 80–90 percent of those diagnosed as having MS have the relapsing and remitting form (RRMS). After about ten years (without treatment), about half of this number (45 percent of total) commence a downward progression without remission, this is known as the secondary progressive form of multiple sclerosis (SPMS). However, like many other chronic illnesses, the course of MS is unpredictable, and the experience of living with the illness is characterised by uncertainty for both patients and carers.

In 1995, even before they were licensed for use in the UK, the question of how the introduction of this new drug treatment for MS for use with the NHS should be managed was concentrating minds within the Department of Health. This was because given the numbers of patients with MS in Britain who would be suitable candidates for treatment, there was a real fear that costs would spiral out of control. At the time one estimate was that if all the patients with RRMS were treated with beta interferon, the cost to the NHS would be equivalent to 10 percent of its total drugs budget (New, 1996). The Conservative government, politically committed as it was to the setting of health spending limits, moved to intervene directly in order to control the costs that would be incurred if clinicians were allowed to prescribe this new treatment for MS without regulation. The NHS Executive subsequently issued a set of guidelines in 1996 addressing the question of who could prescribe the drug, specifying that this could only be regionally-based consultant neurologists and not local GPs. However, resentment built amongst MS patients' groups denied access to the drug, and pharmaceutical companies denied the opportunity to sell and profit from the drug they had expensively developed. Thus, when the work programme for the newly established NICE was first set out in August 1999, coincidentally or not, beta interferon was listed as one of the first technologies to be appraised (NHS Executive, 1999).

The Appraisal Committee examining beta interferon took evidence from the interested parties (MS patient groups and charities, consultant neurologists, the Royal College of Nursing, and the pharmaceutical companies concerned with the development of the drug) in May 2000 and produced a provisional appraisal of the evidence (PAD) by July 2000. However, this preliminary confidential decision (because of the implications for the share price of the drug technology under appraisal) was leaked to the BBC News in June 2000, the subsequent publicity given to the decision not to recommend the treatment produced a widespread outcry from MS patient groups and others. This confidential decision-making process was subsequently revised in February 2001 in order to avoid just these types of accusations in future. The interest groups subsequently appealed against this decision. The NICE Appeal Panel met in November 2000 to discuss the points put to them by the appellants and upheld the complaint that the Appraisal Committee had failed to explain the basis of its argument that beta interferon was not cost-effective, and that it had not compared the cost of treatment with alternative uses of current resources. The Appraisal Committee was told to reconsider the evidence, and to review the particular economic model it had used to appraise cost-effectiveness (NICE, 2000a). Following this judgement the Institute commissioned a 'further economic modelling' of beta interferon.

NICE published its final 'technology appraisal guidance' report (NICE, 2002a) in February 2002, setting out in detail the reasons for the decision not to recommend beta interferon. The report is of interest because it has subsequently provided a template for NICE appraisals of drug technologies. The report shows that the Appraisal Committee did not attempt to challenge the findings of the published clinical trials that were broadly supportive of the clinical effectiveness of these drugs; rather the Committee chose to concern themselves primarily with the issue of cost-effectiveness utilising its revamped yet uncertain economic model. The appraisal concluded that beta interferon was not a cost-effective treatment because it fell outside the 'Cost per QALY Gained' (CQG) ratio used to assess previously appraised disease-modifying treatments. Finally, in coming to its decision not to recommend the use of beta interferon, the Appraisal Committee stated that they were following the directions set out by the Secretary of State for Health, which required NICE to balance the degree of clinical need of people with a disease condition with the benefits and costs of treatment, as well as with the 'efficient use of NHS resources' (NICE, 2002a: 9).

However, just two days prior to the NICE announcement it was revealed in the press that the Department of Health had been in consultation with the pharmaceutical companies concerned with the manufacture of beta interferon drugs and had drawn up what was termed a 'risk-sharing scheme'. This agreement would see the NHS funding the prescribing of beta interferon, but after an agreed timespan an assessment would be made to see if the drug was cost-effective for each patient based on the use of QALYs. If the net cost of the treatment outweighed the expected clinical benefit, then the cost of the drug to the NHS would be 'adjusted' by manufacturers on the basis of a 'sliding scale'. Thus, when the Appraisal Committee made its final announcement that it would not be recommending the use of beta interferon for the treatment of RRMS, the authority attached to this guidance had already been critically undermined.

The obvious question that arose from this development was why did the Department of Health choose to ignore the guidance of its own advisory body about the cost-effectiveness of beta interferon? The Department of Health (DoH, 2002) subsequently argued that the risk-sharing scheme was introduced to confirm the cost-effectiveness of these treatments through establishing a cohort of patients who would be monitored at regular intervals; thus giving the scheme the veneer of a clinical trial. Nevertheless, the way in which the scheme was structured was strongly criticised for being 'scientifically unsound' (Sudlow and Counsell, 2003). That the risk-sharing scheme largely failed to meet many of the criteria that are generally acknowledged as necessary for a scientifically designed randomised control trial almost certainly reflects the fact that it was introduced primarily for reasons of political expediency in the face of a vociferous campaign mounted by an alliance of MS patients, pharmaceutical companies, as well as the medical profession.

The risk-sharing scheme came into effect in late 2002 and imposed a statutory obligation upon local Health Authorities and Trusts to fund the prescribing of beta interferon for all eligible patients. The advice from the Department of Health to Trusts was that they, '... should regard funding for the scheme in the same way as positive NICE recommendations' (DoH, 2002). In return, the manufacturers agreed to marginally reduce the costs of the drug to the NHS in order to bring it nearer the target NICE set for treatment cost per QALY.[2] However, more than five years after the introduction of the scheme the costs of any treatment failures have not been recouped from the manufacturers, not least because the data from the scheme has yet to be published (as of late 2007). In the meantime, new drug technologies for the treatment of MS are now being rolled out and will eventually supersede beta interferon as the recommended treatment for RMMS.

This case study illustrates the extent to which the New Labour government was prepared to go in order to pursue its cost-effectiveness rationality. That point was reached at the moment when a drug treatment that was acknowledged to be clinically effective was to be denied to patients with MS, and the profits of the manufacturers threatened. Ultimately, the government did recoil from the logical consequences of its own cost-effectiveness ideology and imposed a compromise solution (Crinson, 2004).

After eight years of systematically weighing up the costs and benefits of health technology, NICE has actually so far made very few recommendations to exclude interventions that it has been asked to appraise. Although it has recommended the use of cheaper forms of treatment where more expensive ones were judged to provide little or no extra benefit, its recommendations have so far affected only a very small percentage of total NHS spending per annum. It has been argued that in net terms, NICE's guidance to date has been cost-increasing rather than cost-saving for the NHS (Appleby and Harrison, 2006). It has also been noted that there has been a general dominance of the clinical–economic discourse of cost and clinical effectiveness over more qualitative evidence in its appraisal process, which are often seen as supplicatory by the Institute (Milewa and Barry, 2005).

ACTIVITY

Read the paper by Sheldon.T et al., – *What's the evidence that NICE guidance has been implemented? Results from a national evaluation using time series analysis, audit of patients' notes, and interviews. British Medical Journal* (2004) vol. 329: 999. This paper is free to download at www.bmj.com (use search menu).

  This paper has a self-explanatory title, and is a good example of academic research that seeks to evaluate policy implementation. Based on your reading of this paper and the material presented within this chapter, write down your own conclusions about the relative effectiveness of NICE as a regulatory body responsible for providing guidance on new clinical treatments.

The other major 'arm's length' regulatory body, the Healthcare Commission (launched in 2004), is a reconstituted body that took on the responsibility of CHI for checking standards of the care and reviewing the performance of local healthcare organisations. However, it has a much wider remit than the CHI. The Healthcare Commission conducts annual 'health checks' of all healthcare delivery organisations including the NHS, local authority and private sector providers focusing on promoting healthcare performance, public safety, and promoting improvements in public health in England and Wales. This information is made publicly available and includes the production of a rating (no longer based on stars) for each NHS trust in England. It is also responsible for the second stage of the NHS complaints procedure, carrying out independent reviews of complaints. It is probably too early in the life of the Healthcare Commission to assess its success in meeting its wide-ranging remit. However, there is now evidence that the impact of arm's length monitoring and inspection has not necessarily had the desired impact on the performance of local healthcare organisations that has been claimed for it by the Department of Health; this is discussed below.

In addition to the development of the regulatory and inspection agencies, NICE and CHI, the third element outlined in *The NHS Plan* (DoH, 2000b) designed as a long-term strategy to raise quality standards through the setting of measurable goals to be achieved within designated time frames were the National Service Frameworks (NSFs). Since 1999, the Department of Health has established NSFs for ten defined service or care group users (coronary heart disease; cancer; older people; paediatric intensive care; mental health; diabetes; long-term conditions; renal services; children; and chronic obstructive pulmonary disease). When the new General Medical Services contract for GPs came into operation in 2003 it incorporated a Quality and Outcomes Framework (QOF) that identifies clinical indicators and targets drawn from the NSF standards and other recommended interventions which Primary Care Organisations are now required to meet. The relative performance of an individual Primary Care Organisation in meeting each of these indicators attracts points on a sliding scale that are then converted into payments. Meeting the NSF standards within primary care has thus in effect become an incentivised process for GPs (the implications of this for the doctor–patient relationship were discussed as a case study in Chapter 3).

ORGANISATIONAL CULTURE AND THE MEASUREMENT OF PERFORMANCE WITHIN THE NHS

Although the organisational structures associated with the PAF are inextricably linked to outcome measurements, evidence of such structures being the sole driver of performance is rare. Policy theorists described as 'neo-institutionalists' emphasise the 'relative autonomy' of state institutions and organisations from day-to-day political and economic demands. This approach (discussed in relation to the 'new institutionalism' in Chapter 2) focuses on the ability of state actors (top civil servants, senior managers of local health and social care organisations, and the health professional groups) to use these institutional powers to maintain their own sectional and professional interests. From this perspective, an analysis of NHS performance assessment systems must move beyond a description of strategic policy towards practical operational issues, in order to take account of the influence of competing policy actors and the pre-existing 'culture' of that organisation. This assessment is increasingly understood by central government itself. The Department of Health now recognises that 'cultural change' is a necessary 'primary driver' of improvement in the performance of the NHS. This view reflects an acknowledgement that structural changes designed to improve performance have, in the past, often failed to effect changes in the 'informal structure' or culture of the organisation. As H. Davies (2002) has argued, culture acts 'as a kind of social and normative glue' which defines what is 'acceptable and legitimate' within the organisational context.

However, the assumption of a link between a change in organisational culture and performance is one that in practice is difficult to empirically assess. Scott et al.'s (2003) review of ten studies which explicitly examined the relationship between culture and performance within healthcare organisations, concluded that if a relationship existed at all it was 'multiple, complex and contingent'. This conclusion may, in part, reflect the methodological difficulties that are associated with defining and operationalising 'culture' and 'performance', both being constructs that are conceptually and practically distinct. These authors go on to acknowledge that there are many competing conceptualisations: they themselves define organisational culture as those meanings and values that are shared by group members within the organisation and given expression in their working practices. They argue that culture operates at different levels within an organisation, from the observable in relation to particular patterns of behaviour, to less visible beliefs and values, which shape the working assumptions used by staff in their everyday interactions. These assumptions become 'cultural' in the sense that they are seen to assist the group managing everyday problems within the organisation and so are taught to new members as being the correct way to respond.

In relation to the definition of 'performance', Scott et al. (2003) argue that whilst it is often presented as a 'hard-nosed' concept in practice it is, '… less an objective phenomenon and more … something that is both negotiated and socially mediated' (2003: 110). As an example of these local organisational processes, Bevan and Hood (2006) have argued that the use of healthcare targets has resulted in 'gaming' by local healthcare trusts, so that when reported performance meets the national targets, neither government nor the public can distinguish between the following four outcomes:

- All is well : performance has been exactly as desired (whether measured or not);
- The organisation's performance has been as desired where performance was measured, in the domains where performance was not measured the potential for poor performance is high;

- Although performance against targets is good, the activities of local organisations have been at variance with the substantive goals behind these targets (hitting targets but missing the point!);
- Targets have not been met, but this has been concealed by the way in which the data was reported or by outright fabrication (Bevan and Hood, 2006: 421).

Bevan and Hood (2006) concluded that assessing performance by means of an audit system reliant on statistical data rather than regular inspection visits by the Healthcare Commission is open to systematic gaming by local organisations fearful of the outcomes that follow poor performance. This conclusion is also supported by Mannion, Davies and Marshall's (2005) study of the perceptions of local managers' and senior clinicians' within six acute hospital trusts of the 'cultural shift' that had occurred within their organisation following the public reporting of the hospital's performance. This study found a largely negative response amongst these senior staff to the star-ratings system, with a number of 'dysfunctional' consequences seen as arising from the introduction of this method of measuring performance. Many of the clinicians reporting that their clinical priorities had been altered to meet short-term targets. Local managers gave examples of gaming employed by their organisation to improve their measured performance in order to mitigate the perceived unfairness of a ratings system that did not take into account local contingencies, such as the difference between operating in a new purpose-built hospital or a former workhouse, that were beyond their control. However, the influence of the NPM was also present in that hospital managers were able to use these public reports of performance to bring about changes in traditional ways of working; '... as a lever to influence staff behaviour (sometimes positively to motivate them and sometimes negatively to bully them)' (Mannion et al., 2005: 23). Chang's (2007) empirical study of the impact of performance measures similarly found that the use of the PAF by local healthcare managers was primarily 'symbolic and ceremonial' and not used for rational performance improvement. Chang concluded that the PAF gave local managers legitimacy because its use demonstrated a commitment to national goals, but it had little actual impact on improving those aspects of performance valued by local NHS managers. Finally, Exworthy et al.'s (2003) study of the impact of performance indicators on GPs professional identity and clinical autonomy demonstrated the way in which performance management can turn into a battle of strength with the medical profession. However, it should be noted that following the introduction of the incentivised GP contract in 2003 many of the objections cited by GPs in the study may have subsequenctly been mollified.

DECENTRALISING DECISION-MAKING: AN ORGANISATIONAL MODEL FOR THE NHS?

One of the key elements of New Labour's strategy of governance within the NHS is the decentralising of power and decision-making to local healthcare trusts. This is seen as a necessary requirement in order to meet the political commitment of achieving a greater responsiveness to local health needs, widening patient choice, and promoting organisational efficiency. The underlying premise is that decentralisation will 'shorten' the bureaucratic hierarchical structure and so allow greater flexibility for local trust managers and health professionals, which will create the basis for a 'bottom-up' improvement in organisational performance.

Decentralisation as a principle is not new in public policy, and British governments since the 1970s have rarely openly sought to defend the existence of 'command and control' centralised state mechanisms; although the reality is that none sought to dismantle such mechanisms, whatever the political rhetoric. Previous Conservative governments, particularly those led by Margaret Thatcher, made great play of their commitment to 'cutting back bureaucracy' and 'simplifying' government. One of the first health policy documents produced by the Thatcher government when it came to power, *Patients First* (DHSS, 1979b), placed great stress on the need to decentralise and reduce 'interference' from the centre in health needs decision-making. The creation of the 'internal market' in healthcare with its purchaser/provider split and the development of 'self-governing' trusts (DoH, 1989a) was seemingly a major shift in the decentralisation of power. In retrospect, however, most commentators are agreed that on the contrary these reforms established a clear line-management system that Stalin himself would have envied (Timmins, 1996: 511). Indeed, Klein (2001: 182) argues that it was only at this point in its then 50-year history that the NHS became a national service, with lines of accountability running directly to the centre, in the person of the Secretary of State for Health.

New Labour's commitment to decentralisation appears to be more concrete, devolving power from Westminster to the Scottish Parliament, and to the National Assemblies in Wales and Northern Ireland. A commitment to reducing bureaucratic control from the centre and restoring autonomy to health professionals within a decentralised NHS was a key feature of *The New NHS: Modern, Dependable* (DoH, 1997a); and given greater detail in *The NHS Plan* (DoH, 2000b). Nevertheless, these strategy documents, together with the commissioned Wanless Report (2002) into the future funding of the health service, do also have strong centralising tendencies particularly around the management of changes in primary care. Since 2003 decentralising initiatives have included 'earned autonomy' for local trusts (discussed above), the devolution of the bulk of the NHS budget to the PCTs (albeit within strict terms of reference), proposals to encourage high-performing trusts to apply for Foundation Hospital status, and the promotion of the process of widening patient choice (discussed in Chapter 9).

These decentralising initiatives came at the same time as the Department of Health was establishing a more centralised regulatory performance framework. Many commentators (see Newman, 2001) have noticed that there is an obvious tension between the commitment to decentralisation and the 'modernisation' agenda which aims to achieve uniformity in standards, central accountability and performance monitoring across what is a *national* health service. Klein (2001: 106) has also made the point that decentralising decision-making power and giving greater autonomy to local healthcare organisations is always going to be problematic in a national health service funded through direct taxation. Peckham et al. (2006), in their review of decentralisation processes within publicly-funded healthcare systems, have argued that these apparent contradictions reflect a simultaneous process of centralisation and decentralisation, in which local performance outcomes are set centrally ('outcome centralisation') and if met locally lead on to greater autonomy from centralised inspection and financial strictures ('process decentralisation'). Peckham et al. (2006) also make the assertion that there is often a distinct lack of clarity associated with the use of the term 'decentralisation,' which in turn makes it difficult to treat it as a uni-dimensional independent variable in evaluation studies. So for example, in the case of the recent history of the NHS, decentralisation has been presented as a means to achieve better local adherence to organisational performance outcomes, improved internal organisational processes (flexibility, innovation, staff morale, responsiveness, greater public accountability), and as a means to achieving greater equity and access to services for patients (discussed in Chapter 9).

Although Peckham et al. (2006: 118) acknowledge that the evidence linking health outcomes and decentralisation is weak, contingent and limited, overall they conclude that what evidence there is does not support the assumption much favoured by contemporary organisational theory, that decentralised healthcare systems have improved outcomes for patients, more efficient coordination and communication processes, and deliver improvements in organisational performance. The authors go on to argue that the evidence would suggest that there is no optimal size for decision-making or undertaking performance functions within organisations. Although there is some evidence to support the view that decentralisation may lead to more responsive services for specific groups, '(t)hese gains may need to be balanced against other measures of performance such as economies of scale and equity' (Peckham et al., 2006: 120). The authors conclude their review by asserting that one of the major problems associated with the incorporation of decentralisation as a policy strategy for the NHS is that it is based on a series of assumptions about its positive impact on organisational performance which are not supported by evidence nor theory (Peckham et al., 2006: 126).

SUMMARY

The 'performance' of public services, including the NHS, has become a major political concern over the past two decades. Although tempered by an increased concern under the New Labour government with 'quality' and 'standards', the notion of 'performance' within public organisations focuses predominantly on the economic and efficient use of resources. As John Clarke has argued, this particular conception of performance sustains a discourse that emphasises the value, authority and autonomy of managers, and continues the 'competitive' framing of service delivery first initiated under the previous Conservative government in the form of league tables, benchmarking, star-ratings and 'successful' or 'failing' local delivery organisations (Clarke, 2004: 131). Nevertheless, constructing a performance management framework within the NHS has been an immensely complex task given the multitude of system objectives and the diversity of healthcare provision. There is great potential for a lack of coherence and disjuncture between national strategic goals, the activities of the regulatory 'arm's length' bodies such as NICE and the Healthcare Commission, and local organisational priorities. However, there are also important questions about the 'leadership capacity' of top officials within the NHS Executive and the Department of Health to challenge entrenched organisational cultures that are resistant to change and scrutiny.

FURTHER READING

Department of Health (2004) *The NHS Improvement Plan: Putting People at the Heart of Public Service*. Cmnd 6268. London: The Stationery Office. Available at: www.dh.gov.uk/en/Publicationsandstatistics/Publications/PublicationsPolicyAndGuidance/DH_4084476

Peckham, S., Exworthy, M., Powell, M. and Greener, I. (2005) Decentralisation, centralisation and devolution in publicly funded health services: decentralisation as an organisational model for health-care in England. Report to the NHS NCC-SDO research and development programme. Available at: http://www.sdo.lshtm.ac.uk

Walshe, K. (2003) *Regulating Healthcare: A prescription for improvement*? Maidenhead: Open University Press.

9 A PATIENT-LED HEALTH SERVICE? CHOICE, EQUITY AND THE SUPPLIER MARKET

CHAPTER CONTENTS

- Background: a framework for healthcare reform
- Commissioning and the expanding role of the 'supplier' market
- 'Empowering' the service-user?: the 'choice agenda' and the 'demand-side' reforms within the NHS
- Issues of equity in access and treatment
- Summary

BACKGROUND: A FRAMEWORK FOR HEALTHCARE REFORM

Since coming to power in 1997, the New Labour government has been heavily committed to the 'modernising' of the NHS (DoH, 2000b). However, to see this strategy as following something approximating a physical trajectory (senior civil servants often use the term, 'direction of travel') towards a clearly defined set of goals for a national health service in the twenty-first century, would be to accept the rhetoric of government at face value. Even a relatively superficial socio-political analysis of New Labour's health strategy over the past decade reveals a number of what might be termed policy 'strands', resulting in often conflicting demands on the organisation. Many of these policy initiatives have been discussed in the preceding chapters, and include the drive towards raising organisational performance through target and standard-setting to be delivered by forms of 'new managerialism', the largely rhetorical commitment to 'decentralisation' of power and decision-making within the NHS, as well as the imposition of top-down forms of regulation over the activities of professionals and local health delivery organisations.

Now in its third term of office, the New Labour government has asserted that its initial organisational reforms were aimed at overcoming the service inefficiencies that it had inherited and which had led to long waiting lists for treatment and a demoralised workforce. It had to ensure that the new structural mechanisms (described above) were in place in order that the large increases in funding and investment in the NHS that it was committed to would deliver actual improvements in the quality of patient services. Having achieved these organisational reforms and delivered on its investment promises the government felt able to move towards a series of reforms that would deliver its vision of an NHS that was 'patient-led' rather than 'politician-led' (DoH, 2005a).

The ideology of prioritising 'patient choice' and decision-making can be found within Health White Papers that stretch back over two decades to the early years of the previous Conservative administration. New Labour's proposals for this shift in focus in the organisation of the health service were first set out in a White Paper, *The NHS Improvement Plan* (DoH, 2004c), which had as its sub-title the stirring phrase, 'Putting people at the heart of public services'. The Secretary of State for Health at the time, John Reid, set out the 'vision' of a patient-led NHS in the Preface to the White Paper in the following terms; 'An NHS which is fair to all of us and personal to each of us by offering *everyone* the same access to, and the power to choose from, a wide range of services of high quality, based on clinical need, not ability to pay' (DoH, 2004c: 6 – emphasis in original).

The NHS Improvement Plan (DoH, 2004c) sets out a persuasive case for the shift towards a 'patient-led' service, although it is rather less than forthcoming on how this is to be achieved in practice (these details were to come in a document produced by the NHS Chief Executive in the following year – DoH, 2005a). The key assertion of the document is that achieving the goal of a 'patient-led' service requires the organisation to provide and facilitate greater patient 'choice' (it should be noted that 'choice' is a Department of Health policy for England and does not apply to patients who are registered in Northern Ireland, Scotland or Wales). Choice is to come about in four main ways. First, it will be achieved by 'empowering' patients so that they themselves are able to have greater personal control and therefore be in a position 'to call the shots about the time and place of their care' (DoH, 2004c: 9). Second, the building of a new 'supply' market which will allow patients to choose from any healthcare provider, yet all treatment procedures will continue to be paid for by the NHS. It is planned that up to 15 percent of these treatment procedures carried out on behalf of the NHS will be provided by the 'independent' sector (DoH, 2004c: 10). Two key supply-side initiatives were also proposed, the first of these was the creation of Foundation Trusts. These would be trusts (acute hospitals and mental health trusts) who, having met the star performance criteria set by the Department of Health, would be given autonomous status within the NHS and so able to compete as independent providers of care. The other key initiative was the enabling of 'independent' (private sector) providers to compete for contracted clinical services for NHS patients.

The third vehicle that was proposed as a means for the promotion of patient choice was the development of a more extensive electronic information system that would enable patients to become more actively involved in their own health. This was to include the expansion of the services to patients available through NHS Direct, the creation of an electronic booking system so that patients could arrange appointments when it suited them, and the rolling out of an electronic patient record (EPR) with the aim of enabling rapid access by healthcare professionals, so ensuring a comprehensive and seamless service for patients; this would also act to reduce the risk of errors in treatment. Lastly, a new organisational payment mechanism termed 'Payment by Results' (PbR) was introduced in order to facilitate the goal of 'money following the patient'. This system, in which the provider of care is paid a fixed amount for each patient procedure it carries out, was designed to raise the quality of services and 'support the exercise of choice by patients'; this system was to become fully operational by 2008 (DoH, 2004c: 11).

Implementing this bundle of initiatives, intended to initiate a strategic realignment within the health service, from a centrally directed service to a patient-led one, has not been a straightforward process. Delivering 'patient choice' required a higher degree of complementarity between the range of proposals as originally set out in the Improvement Plan, and this was the function of a document produced for local and national health service managers by the Department of Health the following year, with the self-explanatory title *Creating a Patient-led NHS – Delivering the NHS Improvement Plan* (DoH, 2005a). A flavour of the Department of Health policy thinking in this document comes across in the following statement: 'Regulatory, institutional and cultural barriers limit choice, stifle innovation and deter possible new provider. These barriers also create discontinuity for patients when organisations fail to join up around the patient' (DoH, 2005a: para 2.29). The implicit message was that if the goal of patient choice were to be achieved, a new market of providers needed to be allowed to flourish, free from traditional health service constraints. These constraints are identified as follows : '..(t)he hierarchical traditions of the NHS with professional divides and bureaucratic systems and inflexible processes (DoH, 2005a: para 4.4). These barriers to choice were to be overcome primarily through a reworking of the pre-existing system of commissioning.

Primary care practices and PCTs were now to have a much more direct role in commissioning services at the local level so as to enable patients to have a wider choice of provision to meet their healthcare needs. New forms of multi-disciplinary working between health and social professionals were to be promoted, together with the application of the new information technologies such as the electronic 'Choose and Book' service, together with the ongoing establishment of the Electronic Patient Care Record. These developments it was envisaged would enable patients to have more choice when making appointments to see their GP, as well as providing the information to enable them to make their choices about treatment from at least four providers (DoH, 2005a: para 5.22). Since January 2006, all eligible patients referred by their GP for elective care should have been offered clinically appropriate choices from a list of four or more providers commissioned by their PCT. It was envisaged by the Department of Health that the rolling out of these ICT developments (with an initial target date for the end of 2005), backed up by a new system of financial incentives for staff and organisations (such as the new G P contract, and the PbR system) would allow much greater flexibility of service provision, thus facilitating patient choice. As of February 2008, the 'Choose and Book' service was being used for over 45 percent of NHS referral activity from GP surgery to first outpatient appointment, with over 85 percent of all GP practices using the service to refer their patients to hospital, while the Electronic Prescription service (EPS) was used for over 17 percent of daily prescription messages (NHS *Connecting for Health* website – accessed February 2008).

The Department of Health framework for the reform of the NHS (*Health Reform in England: Update and Next Steps* – DoH, 2005b) is presented in diagrammatic form as Figure 9.1 below. This diagram demonstrates the reorientation of the policy direction towards a more consumerist and market-led solution to the achievement of the goal of a 'patient-led' health service in which the 'service-user' becomes more 'assertive and influential' (DoH, 2005b). In this reform document, the conception of market supply and demand that is found in classic economics is meshed with a regulatory approach to improving organisational performance with the goal of achieving a greater responsiveness to the needs of patients. The remaining sections of this chapter examine the notions of 'supply' and 'demand' in relation to healthcare delivery.

COMMISSIONING AND THE EXPANDING ROLE OF THE 'SUPPLIER' MARKET

The process of 'commissioning' provider health services is often differentiated in the health policy literature from 'purchasing' and 'contracting'

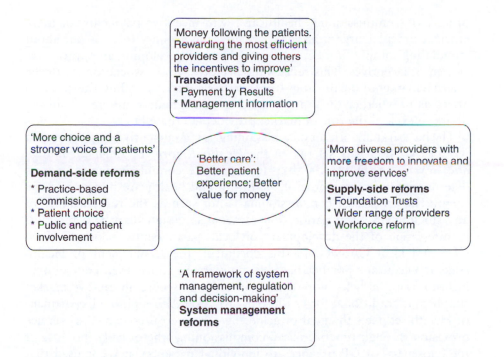

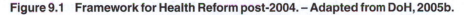

Figure 9.1 Framework for Health Reform post-2004. – Adapted from DoH, 2005b.

(although in practice these terms are often blurred) by reference to the fact that the latter two organisational processes are much narrower in scope than commissioning. From this perspective, purchasing is conceived as being mainly concerned with buying health services from healthcare facilities. Whilst 'contracting' is even more narrowly defined, as the negotiated agreement or tender between purchasers and providers about the services they will provide in return for payment. On the other hand, the process of commissioning involves the development and planning of a national health strategy and its implementation, both through purchasing health services and through influencing a range of organisations to participate in creating the conditions to enhance the population's health; this can only be a function of the public sector (Duran et al., 2005).

The key question that arises from the Department of Health's vision of a patient-led NHS is, whether it is any more deliverable through the structural and organisational strategy of commissioning currently being implemented, than was the case for the Conservative Government's 'Working for Patients' reforms that were to be delivered through the creation of a purchaser-provider 'internal market'? At the heart of the New Labour government strategy is the expansion of the provider or 'supplier' market through this process of 'commissioning' healthcare, with incentive payments for more efficient provider organisations. Formally, the primary focus is not about stimulating competition between providers but developing an appropriate system of incentives. This reflects the need to avoid associations with the internal market of the previous Conservative government. But, the question arises as to whether there are more than just semantic differences in the desire to expand the role of market providers in the NHS.

The basic framework for commissioning as it is currently being developed within the NHS was set out in the *Health Reform in England: update and next steps* (DoH, 2005b). Here, practice commissioning is seen as determining how the whole of the health and healthcare budget is to be spent. The process of commissioning is not seen as the responsibility of any single NHS organisation, but rather it is designed to be a practical manifestation of the development of local 'partnerships' between PCTs, GPs, and local CASSRs. In this document, the Department of Health seeks to encourage practice-based commissioners to use their control over health service budgets more flexibly in order to secure alternative market suppliers to traditional forms of NHS provision.Although the Department of Health set itself the goal of achieving a 'universal coverage' of service provision through practice-based commissioning (rhetorically, because of the 'closeness' of GP practices to individual patients), it recognised that practices required the logistical support of PCTs (for example, in drawing upon QOF disease data in order to assess whether local prevalence differed from PCT averages which would require focused interventions by a particular practice) to enable them to effectively plan for the overall health needs of a local population. PCTs were thus given the responsibility of holding the commissioning funds (with local practices holding indicative rather than real budgets in the short to medium term) and contracts for local providers (hospital trusts, and other voluntary and independent sector organisations) on behalf of their local practices. This decision follows from the fact that PCTs are publicly accountable for the use of NHS resources. As the implementation document acknowledges; '(E)ffective commissioning will depend greatly on the quality of the relationship between PCTs and their local General Practices' (DoH, 2005b: 28).

As of early 2008, the Department of Health remains committed to the 'direction of travel' of a practice-based system of commissioning to meet the health service requirements of the population. However, the timescale for a full implementation of this 'supply-led' reform has had to be constantly updated. This is partly because of issues associated with the delay in implementing the National Programme for Information Technology in the NHS (NPfIT) which is seen as essential for the sharing of information necessary for the local commissioning of services (House of Commons Health Select Committee, 2007). There are also practical questions about the clarity of the vision for delivery of patient-led services through the means of practice-based commissioning. Questions continue to remain about whether the government is fully committed politically to developing a supplier market within the NHS. Expanding the role of commissioning logically requires PCTs to cease being primarily a provider of healthcare, becoming rather a purchasing organisation coordinating and regulating new suppliers to enable them to enter 'the market' without the 'permission' implied by the system of centrally run contracts which has pertained up until now (King's Fund, 2006: 7). This would mean the role of the Department of Health eventually being confined to defining the broad priorities for healthcare and setting the regulatory frame, but with no involvement in the day-to-day management of the health service (King's Fund, 2006: 11). Alternatively, the Department of Health may see commissioning as a process that uses the threat of competition from the independent sector in order to provide a stimulus to raising the performance of NHS organisations. There are precedents for this latter approach. The New Labour government has used the private sector in the past to challenge the public sector rather than to create a full supplier market, both in the prison service and in education in relation to the running of local education authorities.

Regulating a provider market in healthcare, as opposed to the delivery of provision, can be seen to require two separate regulatory roles: economic regulation and quality inspection. The former would involve government developing a system of regulation which focused on competition policy (the impact of mergers and acquisitions amongst providers), and the related issue of the implications for service provision of financial and performance failure by market providers. In practice, it would be highly unlikely that the government would want to give up its control over the setting of prices for particular care services as a tool for managing the efficiency of NHS services. Nevertheless, the Department of Health's PbR system (which has taken nearly five years to implement) does not formally utilise 'price' as a mechanism; this is because the new supplier market has been formally designed to promote competition between providers on the basis of quality not price. To this end the government has set a national 'tariff' for clinical treatments based upon national average costs. By adjusting the tariff/price downwards for a particular service/treatment gains in efficiency can in principle be realized. In 2006, although the tariff only increased by 1.5 percent on average, it was increased by up to 5 percent for elective procedures in order to provide an incentive to providers to cut the waiting times (DoH, 2006b).

Although the government remains formally committed to the expansion of the supplier market, the policy of setting a national tariff in order to maintain control over the cost-efficiency of the health service (even when tariffs have been wrongly costed because of inadequate information and the use of crude analytical measures) has laid down an equivocal message to those who would like to see a widening of the supplier market where prices for NHS services were set largely through unregulated market competition. On this point, Paton (2006), in his critique of the role of the 'new market' in the NHS, sees not equivocation, but rather 'good old fashioned command and control' government which has been given 'a premature obituary.' Here Paton (2006) is drawing attention to the existence of a 'visible hand' (the PCT as standard-setter and regulator in the new commissioning system), behind which lies an 'invisible fist' (a continuing control role for government). This command role for the Department of Health is seen to be reflected in the attempt to 'rationalise' what are deemed to be several 'incompatible' policy streams emergent from the 'garbage can' of recent health policy (a reference to March and Olsen's model of decision-making, described in Chapter 3 above). These 'incompatible' streams are as follows: Firstly, the old, pre practice-based commissioning market, based on purchaser contracting; secondly, the 'third way' of local collaboration and 'partnership'; thirdly, 'neo-command and control' based on the Department of Health's performance targets promulgated down 'un-joined-up vertical silos'; and fourthly, the new market of patient choice underpinned 'shakily by PbR' (Paton, 2006: 127).

Whether Paton (2006) is correct or not in his analysis of the government's attempt to 'rationalise the irrational' in health policy, a strategy has emerged which reflects a market bias in service delivery but which also retains important elements of control from the centre. The latter is reflected in the apparent reluctance to allow local practices to have full control over commissioning budgets, a source of deep concern for those (such as Julian Le Grand, see below) who have been advising the Department of Health in the construction of a 'new consumer market' to drive its 'demand-side' reforms of the NHS. The concern of such reformers is that if the decision has been made by government to create a healthcare system based upon market suppliers, why do decisions concerning its implementation continue to be driven by politics? One answer to this question lies in the discussion of the decision-making processes surrounding policy that were outlined in Chapter 3 above; bureaucratic systems do not give up their power lightly.

ACTIVITY

Read the paper by Pollock, A. and Godden, S. – 'Independent sector treatment centres: evidence so far,' *British Medical Journal* (2008) vol. 336 (issue 7641): 421–424. This paper is free to download at www.bmj.com (use search menu).

In this paper Pollock and Godden look at the working of the new supplier market in healthcare provision, focusing on independent sector treatment centres providing elective surgery on behalf of the NHS. The authors look at the evidence for these centres offering value-for-money for the taxpayer as claimed by the government, using the Department of Health's own performance criteria.

Summarise the case presented by Pollock and Godden in support of their claim that Independent treatment centres lack the efficiency and effectiveness claimed for them by the Department of Health.

'EMPOWERING' THE SERVICE-USER?: THE 'CHOICE AGENDA' AND THE 'DEMAND-SIDE' REFORMS WITHIN THE NHS

From the time that Alan Milburn took over from Frank Dobson as Secretary of State for Health in 2001, the promise of greater patient 'choice' and more 'personalised' healthcare services took on a much more prominent place within New Labour health strategy. New Labour's embracing of the 'choice agenda' (as it has become known) is an essential element in the construction of its consumerist model for the reform of public services. As such it represents an important continuity with the public service policies of the Conservative governments of the 1980s and 1990s. As Clarke and Newman (2006) have noted, the 'choice agenda' represents the promotion of a form of popularism (the New Labour government as 'people's champions') rather than being a genuine extension of democratic participation in government; '… in the sense that everyone is, or ought to be, entitled to choice' (Clarke and Newman, 2006: 4). To illustrate this point Clarke and Newman (2006) quote the then Prime Minister, Tony Blair, from a speech he gave to the Fabian Society in 2003:

Extending choice – for the many, not the few – is a key aspect of opening up the system in the way we need. But choice for the many because it boosts equity. It does so for three reasons. First, universal choice gives poorer people the same choices available only to the middle classes. It addresses the current inequity where the better off can switch from poor providers. But we also need pro-active choice (for example, patient care advisors in the NHS) who can explain the range of options available to each patient. Second, choice sustains social solidarity by keeping better off patients and parents within the NHS and public services. Third, choice puts pressure on low quality providers that poorer people currently rely on.

It is choice with equity we are advancing. Choice and consumer power as the route to greater social justice not social division (Blair, 2003).

Here healthcare choice concerning the delivery of a public service and the politics of consumerism are wrapped together by the Prime Minister. Consumerism as a Key Concept in policy analysis is set out below.

KEY CONCEPT: CONSUMERISM

Consumerism as an analytical construct has a particular reading of *power* as residing in the choices exercised by citizens when purchasing and consuming goods and services, from fridges to healthcare. This 'consumer power' is seen as having forged a demand-led market with important consequences for the manufacturing, retailing and service efficiency of market corporations. Consumerism as a construct has been strongly associated over the past two decades with a neo-liberal political discourse that urges an opening up of state health and welfare services to the exercise of service-user choices. It is asserted that the logic of choice driving efficiency in the market when transferred to the public sector will bring about improvements to the quality of services as providers seek to respond to clients/patients needs.

Consumerism as a political critique of the failure of state welfare services, somewhat ironically was first employed by the political left in the 1960s and 1970s to challenge the professional self interests and bureaucratic paternalism that failed to respond to service-users needs. The construct was used to argue for the *rights* of users to greater *participation* in the public service decisions that directly affected their lives. Today, consumerism as a political discourse is less focused on strengthening user 'rights' to public services and more concerned with widening 'choices.'

New Labour's commitment to the 'choice agenda' was given a policy form with the publication (described in detail above) of *The NHS Improvement Plan* (DoH, 2004c). Here it was stated that,

... (r)apid access is not enough. To meet today's expectations, patients need to be able to choose from a range of services that best meet their needs and preferences. Between now and 2008, the NHS will be making the changes which enable patients to personalise their care and for those choices to shape the system and the way that it is run. (DoH, 2004c: para 2.9)

However, choice is a term that can be deployed in many different ways: in healthcare this can include the choice of location of treatment, choice of doctor or other health professionals, or choice of procedures/health interventions (Propper, Wilson and Burgess, 2006). The form of choice introduced following the implementation of *The NHS Improvement Plan*, is primarily choice of location of hospital treatment to be offered by GPs to their patients. The goal is that by the middle of 2008, all patients requiring hospital treatment will have the right to 'a free choice' for elective care from any healthcare provider (in the expanded supplier market), as long as the provider meets NHS standards and within the nationally set treatment tariff (DoH, 2007b).

The prerequisites for patients to be able to take advantage of the opportunities for a widening of choice include the need to extend the provision of information, as well as the necessity of 'empowering' patients, particularly those from 'low income social groups.' The 'HealthSpace' initiative proposed in 2004 was intended to allow individuals to electronically access their medical records and to provide information about their personal preferences via the internet. However, this initiative has been subject to a series of delays. More health information has been made available via the 'NHS Choices' website, the web-based NHS information service launched in June 2007, which includes a wide range of NHS performance data available in the form of hospital 'league tables'. However, this whole process of providing information for patients to make informed choices appears to be highly reliant on what could best be described as a series of technical fixes. It can be argued that it requires rather more than the easy access to information if service-users are to be empowered to make choices about their treatment. Patients have until relatively recently been encouraged to 'comply' with the clinical management of their condition recommended by their doctor. Widening patient choice could potentially counter this medical paternalism and encourage the patient-directed focus in medical consultation (discussed in Chapter 6). However, limiting patient choice just to the time and location of hospital appointments is not going to bring about this change in doctor–patient relationships: 'GPs can still direct patients and control the treatment options that they offer. Patient empowerment cannot happen unless professionals are engaged' (Farrington-Douglas and Allen, 2005: 9).

A comprehensive review of the use of published data as a source of information by patients in the USA showed that it had only a limited impact on consumer treatment decision-making (Marshall, 2002). The lack of interest in, and use of, healthcare provider performance data by patients appeared to be due to difficulties in understanding clinical information because of its complexity, lack of trust in the data, problems with timely access to the information, and a lack of real choices. There is considerably less evidence about the impact of choice available on healthcare consumer behaviour in the UK, and even less from Europe. So, although the drive for choice-based healthcare is unanimously supported by all three major political parties in England, this is not a politics that is highly evidence-based (Propper et al., 2006: 551). One of the few sources of data is the regularly updated National Patient Survey conducted by the Department of Health itself. The results of the survey conducted in September 2007 found that less than half (45 percent) of the patients recalled were being offered a choice of hospital for their first out-patient appointment, while 61 percent were unaware before visiting their GP that they had a choice of hospital for a first hospital appointment. Examining the factors that influenced the choices of hospital for those patients who were offered a choice, found that location or transport considerations were most commonly cited (65 percent). Other frequently cited factors were cleanliness (22 percent), the reputation of the hospital (20 percent), waiting times (20 percent), and quality of care only being cited by 15 percent of the patients (Dixon, 2008).

Establishing a demand market in healthcare for incentivised providers has been the primary driver for the introduction of choice in the NHS. However, the national incentive system of payment by results (PbR) for secondary care providers (hospitals) may actually be working to the limitation of patient choice. The PbR, which applies the national pricing or tariff structure to treatments commissioned by PCTs, actually gives hospitals an incentive not to accept more severely ill patients (known as 'dumping'), or to undertreat such patients (known as 'skimping'), and to attract the less severely ill and overtreat these patients (known as 'cream-skimming'). These incentives are intensified when hospitals are subject to competition based on league tables of performance. The effect may well be to concentrate on the treatment of sicker patients in the high quality teaching hospitals. This effect may be exacerbated by new providers in the supply market who cream-skim the easier-to-treat patients. However, the high quality hospitals which attract high volumes of patients with high severity will inevitable have poorer measured patient outcomes, which in turn will affect their position in the league tables, influencing patient choices (Propper et al., 2006: 553). That is, unless outcome measures can be introduced that reflect real patient severity, which is not the case currently.

It should also be noted that the choice now offered to the purchasers of services (the PCTs) in the new system of practice commissioning is not at all the same thing as patients themselves having real choice. At present there is a blurring of these differences by the Department of Health. If the system of purchaser choice of provider is to operate effectively, the choice available to patients may well have to be restricted; the conflict between these two forms of choice is likely to become more apparent when the commissioning system is fully rolled out (Propper et al., 2006: 554). On this point it should be noted that the US market-based healthcare system is characterised by high payer (insurance company) choice but limited direct patient choice.

ISSUES OF EQUITY IN ACCESS AND TREATMENT

The promotion of the choice strategy raises important questions about equity of access and treatment for the NHS of the future. That is, will those patients who are most in need of healthcare services, the more socially deprived, actually benefit from a greater availability of choice of providers? Here the concept of 'equity' as used in relation to healthcare services is utilised in several ways within the literature.

Equity can refer to the distribution of resources within the healthcare system on the basis of greater healthcare need, the issue of 'rationing' services; or it can relate to the degree to which different social groups are able to access healthcare; or it can also refer to the appropriateness of treatment offered to different social groups in meeting their health needs. While the concept of equity of 'outcome' examines how healthcare interventions differentially benefit social groups with different levels of health need (Goddard and Smith, 2001). Nevertheless, the general usage of the term 'equity' in relation to access to healthcare refers to, '... systematic variations in the experience of individuals and social groups that are regarded as unfair' (Baggott, 2004: 191). The existence of inequity in access to healthcare between social groups can arise from differences in social class, gender, ethnicity or disability. The notion of achieving equity of access to healthcare should also be differentiated from the wider issue of reducing 'inequality' of health outcomes that exist between social groups in Britain today (this issue is discussed in Chapter 11).

Since the 1970s, study after study has reported that the NHS provides a less than equitable service (defined in relation to the 'fairness' criteria cited above). Although the NHS was founded on the principles of healthcare provided free at the point of use according to need, analysis has shown that there is a disproportionate utilisation of the healthcare services by the middle classes relative to their self-reported illness; this outcome has become known as the 'inverse care law' (Tudor-Hart, 1971). More recent studies have confirmed that this process continues. There are geographical and transport inequities (for example in relation to car ownership and living in a rural area) which influence access to services. More significantly there are inequities arising from social differences in the ability to assert health needs relating to familiarity and confidence in accessing the health system. These inequities, '... are compounded by unequal healthcare-seeking behaviours, which often disadvantage people from poorer, less educated backgrounds' (Farrington-Douglas and Allen, 2005: 6).

The rather understated conclusion of one recent study of inequity, which drew on self-reported morbidity data from the annual Health Survey for England, was as follows:

> (A)fter controlling for morbidity in a number of dimensions, more deprived individuals (in terms of income, education and employment) have lower than expected use of health services ... . This implies that there may be an unmet need for healthcare in terms of income, employment and educational deprivation. (Sutton et al., 2002: 89)

This particular study is cited in a report, written by a number of key health policy advisors to the government, together with a number of Department of Health officials, summarising the evidence of the persistence of inequity in the NHS (Le Grand et al., 2003). This review concluded that:

> The confidence and ability to articulate among the middle class, their voice, and their ability to express it, and their networks, are clearly key factors affecting their ability to communicate with GPs and to promote referral onwards to secondary and tertiary care ... We can distinguish two types of disadvantage that lower socio-economic groups experience when using the health service: those that relate to the problems of making first contact with the service, and those that concern the problems they experience once contact has been established. Thus relative to the better off, when ill, the poor either tend not to go to the doctor at all, or to present at a later stage in their illness ... if they do establish contact, they then experience another set of difficulties, which manifest themselves in lower rates of referral (Le Grand et al., 2003: 29).

However, Julian Le Grand, who has been an important influence in the development of New Labour's health strategy, uses the evidence of inequity to support his essentially pro-market case for wider choice. His position rests on the assumption that:

> Empowering all patients to make informed choices about their care could equalise the advantage the middle class patients currently exercise through their voice and connections. Higher quality and more tailored information delivered to patients at the time they need it could address the 'inverse information law'. (Le Grand et al., 2003: 30).

This is the argument that extending choice to active consumers of healthcare widens equity. However, a strong case can also be made on the basis of the same evidence that widening choice would only serve to deepen differential access to healthcare services.

John Appleby, chief economist at the King's Fund, in outlining the results of a study by his think tank (commissioned by the Department of Health) into social group differences in treatment choices has argued that; '(T)here is a parallel with schools with middle classes tending to gravitate towards what they perceive as the better schools. If this happens in healthcare we could see potentially a widening of health and health inequalities between those with formal education qualifications and those without' (Reported in *The Guardian*, 31st May, 2006). It is unlikely that the wider social disadvantages which play such an important part in perpetuating inequity can be significantly reduced by a shift in one aspect of health policy alone. The strategy rests heavily on the ability to 'empower' socially disadvantaged patients so that they are able to make informed choices. The consequences of this approach for patients are that with 'empowerment' comes a new set of (individual) responsibilities. But what happens to those individuals who do not make appropriate choices about their health needs, does this represent a system failure or an individual one? The Department of Health has rather belatedly acknowledged the critique of the possible detrimental outcomes on pre-existing health inequities of its choice agenda. In December 2007, it published it initial response to the results of several pilot studies which suggested that, whilst there was no clear evidence to date linking the rolling out of the choice policy with greater inequity, '... there is still the potential that it could do so and work is ongoing to provide support to *all* patients' (DoH, 2007c). To this end, the Department of Health document has now set up an 'equality impact assessment' of its free choice policy.

SUMMARY

The public policy decision-making process models that were outlined in Chapter 3, in particular Lindblom's (1965) incrementalist model ('muddling through' as it became known) or the 'garbage can model' (March and Olsen, 1976; Olsen, 1983), might all be more or less accurate analytical descriptions of what has often appeared to be an extemporaneous attempt by the New Labour government to introduce market forces into the NHS. It is possible to make this claim on the basis of the discussion above concerning the lack complementary between many of the initiatives introduced in order to realise a 'patient-led NHS'. One example of this would be the provision of real patient choice which in principle should obviate the need for commissioners (who are healthcare professionals not patients) to agree contracts with providers, yet both conceptions of choice run alongside each other in the new demand market. This leads to the question: why do governments often appear to be pursuing diverse policy goals contemporaneously?

The application of the incrementalist model would point to the ways in which governments, rather than deciding between apparently competing policy agendas, often choose to incorporate a diversity of political goals. This is an outcome of the policy process that is rarely acknowledged by rational choice public decision-making models. This conclusion also draws attention to the issue of hegemony in policy-making (see Chapter 3), and the degree to which competing groups at the centre of policy-making are able to dominate or control the direction of policy at a particular moment in time.

FURTHER READING

Department of Health (2005a) *Creating a Patient-led NHS – Delivering the NHS Improvement Plan*. London: DoH. Available at: www.dh.gov.uk/en/Publicationsandstatistics/Publications/PublicationsPolicyAndGuidance/DH_4106506

Newman, J. (ed) (2005) *Remaking Governance*. Bristol: Policy Press.

Tudor-Hart, J. (2006) *The Political Economy of Health Care: a Clinical Perspective*. Cambridge: Policy Press.

10 MEETING LONG-TERM HEALTH AND SOCIAL CARE NEEDS IN THE COMMUNITY

CHAPTER CONTENTS

- Introduction
- Background: the health and social care divide
- The development of a 'Community Care' policy
- The organisation of health and social care under the New Labour government
- The role of 'informal carers' in health and social care policy
- Meeting the needs of carers: practicalities and policies
- The state of social care: the need for further reform?
- Summary

INTRODUCTION

Until comparatively recently, the term 'Cinderella services' was used to describe the community or social care services available to the dependent elderly, people with long-term mental illness, people with physical and learning disabilities, and those living with a long-term mental health problem. This term succinctly encapsulates the way in which the complex health and social needs of these groups have historically been marginalised in government health policy.

However, since the early 1990s, this situation has gradually begun to change. Attempts have been made by both Conservative and New Labour governments to coordinate the activities of the NHS and local authorities in developing services that meet the needs of these vulnerable groups. This process has not been without its problems, and this has not been solely due to the rivalries and differences in service delivery culture that have traditionally existed between local authority social services departments and the NHS providers.

The demand for social care provision increases year-on-year. In 2006–07, some 1.77 million adults received packages of care provided by their local councils, who spent £14.2 billion on meeting their health and social care needs. Nevertheless, it is also estimated that an additional £5.9 billion was spent by older people out of their own pockets on their personal care requirements. This indicates that the statutory health and social care services are not fully meeting long-term care needs at a time when the proportion of those aged over 75 is increasing within the population; this is despite large increases in state investment over the past decade. It should also be noted that 80 percent of those using social care services have a long-term healthcare need (DoH, 2006c).

BACKGROUND: THE HEALTH AND SOCIAL CARE DIVIDE

Since the inception of the welfare state in 1945 to the present day, disputes over the proper boundary between the role of the NHS and local council social services have shaped the provision of long-term services for older dependent people and adults with physical and learning disabilities. A major factor in this divide lies in the system of funding available to these two arms of the welfare state. NHS services that are available for the long-term care needs of dependent adults, which include hospital-based care, primary care in the community, and rehabilitation services, are funded by general taxation and continue to remain free at the point of delivery. By contrast, services provided and purchased by local authorities, which include residential homes, day care and domiciliary services, are funded by a mixture of local taxation (household rates up until the 1980s, replaced by the notorious and short-lived community charge or 'poll tax' which every adult in a property aged 18 or over was required to pay, which in turn was replaced by council tax in 1993), central government funding, and means-tested contributions from the users of services.

Before the creation of universal state health and welfare services, those elderly people who required care and support (and who lacked the means to purchase private nursing care) were managed in the large public assistance institutions, often in appalling conditions (frequently in what had been Poor Law workhouses). With the inception of the NHS in 1948 this situation began to change, and long-term healthcare for the 'chronically sick' was now provided in hospital settings free of charge. Older people in need of care because of their social welfare needs were separately provided for in new local authority residential homes. However, demand for local authority residential care soon overtook the places that were available, and this led to disputes between hospitals and local authorities about the appropriate placement of older people, influenced by the different sources of funding available to each. It took central government more than a decade to get around to settling these disputes by issuing a circular to local authorities informing them that they were responsible for the care of the 'senile and infirm' and otherwise incapacitated individuals who were not able to manage without support (Ministry of Health, 1957).

By 1971, local authorities had integrated their various social care functions into Social Services Departments (SSDs), but this did little to resolve the issue of responsibility for the care of the elderly dependent. This situation was exacerbated by the shift in the clinical management of those requiring long-term healthcare that began to occur in the 1970s, which saw a reduction in long-term care beds, quicker discharge procedures and shorter stays in hospital. This shift inevitably led to more demands placed upon council residential care and domiciliary services, and although the role of the hospital services in providing care for elderly dependent people was diminishing, there was no transfer of funding to local authorities. These organisational developments led to '… growing calls for change and reform' (Means, Richards and Smith, 2000), and the instigation of a policy debate as to how health needs were to be distinguished from 'social needs' – defined as a Key Concept below.

KEY CONCEPT: SOCIAL NEEDS

Bradshaw's (1972) taxonomy of needs is frequently cited in the social policy literature as the definitive starting point for any conceptualisation of social need. It has also been utilised to critique the flawed assumption that most people's social needs are met by the welfare state because health and social care services are universal, that is, available to everybody in society according to their need. Here it should be borne in mind that most of the social care services provided by local authorities are means-tested, and many of those provided by the NHS are subject to rationing, and therefore are not in practice universally available to all.

The taxonomy or system of classification developed by Bradshaw identified four possible ways of defining individual needs, set out in a hierarchical form as follows:

- *Felt Need:* when people are conscious of needs but are not explicitly recognised and remains hidden;
- *Expressed Needs:* When needs are known about and become demands;

(Continued)

(Continued)

- *Normative Needs:* Defined according to professional norms or standards;
- *Comparative Needs:* Introduces the notion of social justice. Is one social group getting something others are not?

The taxonomy is built upon the premise that needs are socially constructed, by which it is meant that human social needs are not universal and transcendental, but are a product of a particular society at a particular historical moment. Hence, the concept of social need is frequently contested within health and social policy-making.

Conceptualising social needs as being socially constructed, is recognition that an understanding of social context is essential; an individual is only able to identify a need for something when the provision to meet that need exists. In the context of the existence of a universal system of welfare state provision of social care services, it is the supply of services which conditions the demand for services. Hence, it then becomes possible within social care policy to introduce a set of eligibility criteria which can determine what and what is not a 'need'. This is practically achievable through the utilisation of 'needs assessments' carried out by health and social care professionals.

THE DEVELOPMENT OF A 'COMMUNITY CARE' POLICY

The Community Care Act (1990), which came into operation in 1993, was promoted by the then Conservative government as a 'revolution in social care'. The policy was designed to address the historical failure to prioritise the health and social care needs of the dependent elderly, people with physical and learning disabilities, people with long-term mental health problems, and enable them to live as independently as possible, either in their own homes or in residential care. In examining the political, social and organisational pressures that led the Conservative government to undertake a radical departure in policy direction that required an expansion of state involvement after a decade in power attempting to retrench health and welfare spending, Hadley and Clough (1997) have identified the following five key themes:

- *Growing national resources*: As the national economy expanded following the recession of the mid to late 1980s, there was a new political optimism that social problems could be tackled through increasing public spending.

- *Rising demand – both in terms of demography and expectations*: The increase in both the numbers of those people requiring social care, mainly the dependent elderly with long-term care needs, and in the period of time over which this care now had to be provided because of increased life expectancy. This was seen to be having a detrimental impact both on family support structures as well as the ability of existing local authority services to cope.
- *The strengthening of professionalism*: The increasing numbers and influence of health and social care professionals, with the professional optimism and confidence to urge that personal social care services be expanded in order to effectively manage social care needs.
- *Changing concepts of treatment and good practice*: These include: firstly, advances in drug therapies for mental illness enabling treatment in the community. Secondly, the principle of 'normalisation' – the ideological value that access to health and social services should be equal, regardless of disability or age, and that there should be no separation of service provision for different social groups. Thirdly, the principle of 'integration' – whatever the individual problem or disability, everyone should be able to live in mainstream society. Fourthly, the principle of 'choice' – the needs of clients themselves to be considered in service provision. Finally, a recognition of the importance of living in one's own home or 'homelike' circumstances while receiving care.
- *De-institutionalisation*: The closing of long-stay institutions and asylums.

However important these factors were, probably the single most important factor instrumental in the decision made by the Conservative government in 1988 to set up a Commission to examine the issue of community care (Griffiths, 1988), was the concern with the fiscal consequences of not engaging in a process of reform of services. Throughout the decade of the 1980s, there had been a massive increase in the amount spent by the then Department of Social Security on meeting the residential care fees for the elderly dependent. These fees were met through Income Support payments, which dramatically rose from £10m to £1.8 billion between 1979 and 1991. Indeed, the main terms of reference for the 1988 Commission examining community care was to; '... review the way in which public funds are used to support community care policy and to advise ... on the options for action that would improve the use of these funds as a contribution to more effective community care' (Griffiths, 1988). The Griffiths Report itself was strongly critical of the lack of planning arrangements for health and social care. It recommended that central government take a clearer role, and that local authority SSDs be given an enabling role as the lead agency in community care. SSDs should be able to identify needs and devise packages of care, which should be largely resourced by central government. At the time of the Report's publication, many analysts had severe doubts about the government's willingness to provide the policy leadership recommended by Griffiths. Doubts were also voiced about central government's willingness to give local authorities new powers and responsibilities, given the history of antagonism that existed throughout the 1980s between the Conservative government and local authorities, the vast majority of which were Labour councils. The question then was, would the government accept the thrust of the recommendations which would mean making a policy U-turn on its ideological commitment to reducing the role of the state in welfare planning and provision?

The Conservative government's response came over a year later with the publication of the White Paper, *Caring for People* (DoH, 1989b). Many of the Griffiths recommendations regarding the funding and organisation of social care were accepted, and in particular a new central role was given to the local authority SSDs as 'commissioners' of care services. The Report also sought to promote the development of a 'mixed economy' of care involving both the private and voluntary sectors in provision. Local councils were given the responsibility of jointly planning developing strategies with the local Health Authority to meet local social care needs and produce an annual 'Community Care Plan'; hence the now widely used acronym CASSR – Council with Adult Social Services Responsibilities. Councils and local health authorities were also to devise discharge policies for anyone leaving hospital and in need of care in the community. Under the new legislation, clients were not to be discharged until their care had been planned. One of the most significant changes that the White Paper proposed was to place the identification of need at the centre of the management and service delivery processes. This 'needs assessment' was to be carried out by a professional 'case manager', but users of the service and their carers were also to be directly involved in the process. This new emphasis on 'individual needs-based' social planning marked a fundamental policy shift for the Conservative government given that it had spent much of the previous decade ideologically attacking what it saw as the individual and social 'dependency' historically created by the welfare state. However, the White Paper did depart from the Griffiths Report, in that there was to be no direct link between resource allocation from central government and locally identified needs as expressed in the community care plans (Wistow and Hardy, 1994). This decision was to have fundamental consequences for the implementation of the needs assessment principle.

The basic framework of the White Paper was enacted in 1990 through The NHS and Community Care Act, yet in one important respect there was an important omission, the legislation backtracked on the White Paper's commitment to user rights. There was now to be no statutory requirement for user groups to have an input into their local community care plans, nor any requirement laid upon CASSR's to give reasons for not providing services to individuals. The legislation itself was not implemented until two years after its approval by Parliament (not coming into force until April 1993). The major reason for this delay lay in arguments over funding, and over the designation of responsibilities between the statutory delivery organisations. Powerful interest groups such as the Institute for Health Service Management, the Association of Metropolitan Authorities, the Association of Directors of Social Services and other professional bodies, challenged the Department of Health over what they saw as inadequate funding and lack of clear guidance over planning arrangements for the new system of community care. One of the central issues was the failure to clearly define the difference between health care (the responsibility of the NHS) and social care (the responsibility of CASSRs). This was of course the intractable organisational problem that had so characterised the post-war delivery of health and social care with all its problems of fragmentation which the Community Care Act was meant to overcome. The following example, written at the time of the introduction of the legislation, illustrates what this health and social care divide meant in practice:

> The nurse who enters the client's home to treat a leg ulcer is performing healthcare, by her personal contact with the client, is also conducting an important social function. Equally, many aspects of social care such as personal and house cleanliness, poverty and lack of a social life, have important health consequences. (Healy, 1993)

By 1997, the outgoing Conservative government was able to claim that, four years after the implementation of the Community Care Act, its community care policy had been a success and cited the following statistics for a single week in 1996 – half a million households received 2.5 million hours of home help or home care services, over 800,000 meals delivered, over 600,000 day centre places provided by over 4,600 day centres. Over 1.5 million clients were receiving 'care packages' provided, purchased, or supported by CASSRs following a needs assessment (DoH, 1997b). However, there were other consequences which the government was less willing to acknowledge.

The introduction of a care commissioning role for CASSRs, which was intended to promote a supplier market in social care, also opened up the possibilities for healthcare trusts as well as private companies to bid for provider contracts. It was argued at the time that these changes, '... led to a hardening of attitudes about organisational and professional responsibilities, and less flexibility at the margins between NHS and local authority services' (Local Government Management Board, 1997, cited in

Glendenning and Means, 2004: 442). The consequences were not better collaboration but ongoing boundary disputes between local authorities and local health trusts, particularly in relation to the 'bed-blocking' issue. The latter was said to arise due to the new complex procedures which required a place to be available in a local authority residential or nursing home before an elderly patient requiring support could be discharged from hospital. Given the resource problems endemic to local authorities, there were frequent delays in making these places available. The requirement to develop eligibility criteria, discussed above, followed from the limited resources available to councils in undertaking the responsibility for providing and purchasing community care services, much of which had previously been provided free by the NHS, or through centrally funded income support.

THE ORGANISATION OF HEALTH AND SOCIAL CARE UNDER THE NEW LABOUR GOVERNMENT

The New Labour government inherited a community care system that undoubtedly represented a significant improvement on the fragmented system of service provision for the elderly dependent that had existed the last time a Labour government had been in power (in 1976). Although the new government preferred to use the term 'social care'[1] rather than 'community care', the framework created in 1993 continued to operate very much in its original form.

The emphasis in New Labour health and social care policy has been on improving collaboration, or what have euphemistically become known as 'partnerships' between the public, private and voluntary sectors in the provision of health and social care. This approach was reflected in the proposal to create new integrated organisations called Care Trusts in the NHS Plan (DoH, 2000b), and made mandatory in the Health and Social Care Act of 2001. The objective for these new organisations was to break down the separate funding streams and organisational boundaries between the NHS and local authority SSDs. So that, in theory, Care Trusts as single, multi-purpose legal bodies that can commission and deliver health and social care services for the elderly dependent and other vulnerable groups, could generate greater collaboration and integration of service provision. Care trusts were modelled on NHS Trusts but required local authorities to be fully represented in their governance, to take a share of responsibilities. Those studies which have looked at the single system role of Care Trusts foresaw this initiative as potentially giving the NHS much greater power to focus on the provision of health and social care services around ill-health and treatment (Hudson and Henwood, 2002). In practice, the emphasis placed by the Department of Health on the role of Care Trusts appears to focus more on the reduction of the number of blocked beds in hospitals rather than upon the consideration of the needs of older people *per se*. However, the Care Trust inititive appears to have stalled: as of 2008, there are currently only 11 such trusts in existence across England; this hardly constitutes an endorsement at a local level by PCTs or CASSRs of the single system approach.

The NHS Plan (DoH, 2000b) also announced the publication of a National Service framework (NSF) for Older People (DoH, 2001c). Like all the NSFs, it imposed a series of treatment guideline requirements upon, and regulated the activities of, provider organisations. A key requirement of the NSF for Older People upon PCTs and CASSRs was the introduction of a Single Assessment Process (SAP) as a tangible representation of the 'interface' of joint health and social care assessment and planning for individuals.

The introduction of the SAP also moved on the process of client needs assessment that was first introduced in 1993, requiring, '... (t)he use of a set of standardised domains of need' in devising an individual care package (DoH, 2001a: 31). The introduction of a standardised assessment of need against which interventions could be planned represented a potential diminution of the judgement of social care professionals. But, as a recent critique of this standardised approach to evaluating the long-term care needs of the older client noted; '... (i)t is not the level of physical needs *per se* but how these relate to the level of confidence, family support and availability of publicly funded services, as perceived in 'the crisis', that determines the need for institutional care' (Taylor and Donnelly, 2006: 825). This critique points to the necessity of professionals drawing on their accumulated professional experience when assessing the depth of the 'crisis' that has brought the social care needs of an older person to the attention of the CASSR; this is not a process that is easily captured in an assessment tool. However, for the Department of Health the process of rolling out the SAP is also fundamental to the realisation of its National Programme for Information Technology in the NHS (NPfIT).

The NPfIT's vision for creating shared local records systems was set out in its original specification document for the *Integrated Care Records Service* (NPfIT, 2003) which described the need for integrated clinical information systems across 'the whole care continuum'. The ultimate goal of the Electronic Care Record project is to bring together information from a range of separate and paper-reliant records systems held by GPs, hospitals, and social services together to create a shared electronic record accessible across the local health and social care providers. The timetable set for the delivery and implementation of these electronic systems (which also included the electronic booking service known as 'Choose and Book', and the Electronic Prescription Service) in basic form was the end of 2006, to be in full operation by 2010 (NPfIT, 2003). 'NHS Connecting for Health' came into operation in April 2005, as an agency of the Department of Health, with the responsibility for delivering the NPfIT. However progress has been slow in delivering these information systems, and following the publication of Lord Darzi's interim report, *Our NHS Our Future* (DoH, 2007d) in October 2007, the NHS Chief Executive ordered a review of information use across the health service.

The publication of the White Paper, *Our Health, Our Care, Our Say: a New Direction for Community Services* (DoH, 2006c) signalled, rhetorically at least, an important shift in the organisation and delivery of social care with fewer patients being treated inappropriately in hospital, more services delivered within and near the home with joint health and social care teams assisting people in their daily lives, and more emphasis on preventative care. To this end, the White Paper explicitly defines social care as, '(T)he wide range of services designed to support people to maintain their independence, enable them to play a fuller part in society, protect them in vulnerable situations and manage complex relationships'(DoH, 2006c: 3). However, progress in meeting these goals is dictated by the system of funding of services that is now in place, PCT-directed commissioning. The assumptions underpinning commissioning are that services responsive to patient needs can be delivered through the financial incentives provided by the 'Payment-by-Results' mechanism, which in turn is dependent upon its (inherently) crude system of tariffs (discussed in detail in Chapter 9). However, hospital trusts stand to lose financially if less patients are treated in their institutions, and so have no incentive to work towards the shifting care to more home-based services; the funding system mitigates against the integration of primary and secondary care services in a locality.

THE ROLE OF 'INFORMAL CARERS' IN HEALTH AND SOCIAL CARE POLICY

An important distinction needs to be made between care that is provided *in* the community (carried out by the Healthcare and Social Services), and care *by* the community, or 'informal care' as it is sometimes termed. Informal care is based primarily around kinship obligations that exist between members of the immediate family. The realities of community care policy have, until relatively recently, given these unpaid and untrained family members a largely unacknowledged but pivotal role in the system of health and social care. 'Community' or 'social' care for the vast majority of people who receive care in their own homes has always meant the 'informal care' given to them by their family members (mainly women); some estimates seeing informal care as representing 90 percent of all community care. It was not until 1985 that any large-scale survey of informal carers was carried out by the government; up until that time, research had focused solely on the needs of those requiring physical or social care. It began to be recognised that much more reliable information was required regarding the numbers engaged in caring activities, and so a question was included for the first time in the 2001 census to address this issue. The 2001 census found that there were 5.2 million unpaid carers (one in ten of the population of England and Wales) of which: 68 percent (3.56 million) provided care for up to 19 hours per week; 11 percent (0.57 million) provided care for 20 to 49 hours per week; 21 percent (1.09 million) provided care for 50 or more hours per week (ONS, 2003).

Since the inception of the welfare state in Britain, social care policy has drawn upon a number of normative assumptions about where the responsibilities for such care lie; these are discussed in the following subsections.

THE RELATIONSHIP BETWEEN THE RESPONSIBILITIES OF THE STATE AND THE FAMILY

For the vast majority of those who require support in their own homes, community care has traditionally meant the care given to them by their family members. The introduction of the Community Care Act in 1993 did begin to address the issue of who actually performed these caring tasks. For the first time, there was an acknowledgement by government of its responsibility to provide, through local authorities, domiciliary services, respite care and day care as supplements to family-provided care. Nevertheless, until the development of the 'Carers Strategy' in 2000 (see below), this responsibility was not acted upon. This was despite the fact that the Community Care legislation was quite explicit about defining the role of networks of family and friends in providing care, particularly for the dependent elderly.

A CHANGING CARING ROLE FOR THE FAMILY?

There is a widely held, but essentially moralistic view that the perceived policy 'problem' of the social care needs of groups within society has arisen because as a modern society 'we' no longer take care of our dependent family members. This perspective is predicated on a number of largely false historical assumptions about the extent to which the role and function of the family has changed over the last hundred years. Crucially, the demographic shift towards people living longer has resulted in an increase in the number of dependent elderly people. Interestingly, as long ago as 1911, 5 percent of the elderly population were in some type of institutional care, today that proportion is virtually identical (although absolute numbers are very much higher).

CARING AS 'WOMEN'S WORK'!

Connected to the position that families are taking less responsibility for providing care for their dependent members is a set of assumptions about the changing role and responsibilities of women in society. The sexist assumption that women are expected to undertake the major role in caring for dependants (including pre-school children, children with disabilities, parents and husbands with disabling illnesses, etc.), can still be found in many areas of government health and social policy-making. However, as Marian Barnes (1998) has pointed out, demographic changes, shifts in employment patterns, as well as changes in what are perceived to be acceptable divisions of labour between men and women, have meant that the availability of female family members continuing to take on this role in the future cannot be confidently assumed.

ETHNICITY AND CARING

There has also been a tendency by policy-makers to assume that caring for dependent relatives is not a 'problem' within ethnic minority communities. This reflects stereotypical assumptions regarding the existence of extended families amongst ethnic minorities (particularly Asians), which does not necessarily reflect the reality of the situation. These assumptions have an impact as they can manifest themselves as inequities in formal health and social care provision for ethnic minority groups.

MEETING THE NEEDS OF CARERS: PRACTICALITIES AND POLICY

Whilst informal care carried out by lay carers may reduce the financial cost to the State, the costs, both to the person being cared for and to the carer themselves, are considerable. Caring can impose a heavy financial (despite state allowances), physical and psychological strain on carers. The carer may have had to give up their own career (unpaid care remains undervalued in society), because it is difficult to combine the demands of paid employment with caring responsibilities. Other outside interests may have had to be curtailed in order to meet the needs of the person with the chronic illness. The physical labour involved in meeting the activities of daily living for a relatively immobile person are considerable and are particularly demanding for carers who are likely to be elderly themselves. This can potentially lead to health problems for the carer. Caring relationships are reciprocal, and tensions in pre-existing relationships can arise from the changes in role brought about by the dependency of the recipient of care. Thus, individuals who are now physically dependent on their partner, for example, may feel frustration and anger with their condition which they cannot express in ways that may be possible with a professional carer. In the case of those caring for family members who have a mental health problem, relationships can be strained not just because of the pressure of caring in itself, but because of the ways in which the carers may find themselves socially stigmatised (by association) because they may be seen in some way to be responsible for bringing about the mental health problem in the first place.

In April 1996, the then Conservative government introduced the Carers (Recognition and Services) Act. This piece of legislation represented the first real official recognition of the role of carers and their needs, and as such reflected their pivotal role within the new community care policy. This legislation gave carers (although only those caring for more than 20 hours per week) the right to request an assessment of their own needs (155,000 such assessments were carried out in 1999). Nevertheless, the provision of services to all those carers deemed as being in need was never fully implemented. In February 1999, the Labour government published its national strategy for Carers entitled *Caring about Carers*, a strategy document that represented the outcome of a long consultative process and which was introduced as a 'new, substantial policy package that marks a decisive change from what has gone before' (DoH, 1999b). The national strategy set out a distinct set of objectives for state support to carer; these are outlined below:

- The government acknowledged the value of unpaid care within society, but it was also committed to supporting carers in combining paid employment with their caring responsibilities in order to prevent 'social exclusion'. To this end, employers were to be persuaded of the benefits of having a 'carer-friendly' employment policy.
- Carers were to be informed and consulted about any decision-making concerning those they care for.
- Health professionals were encouraged to consider the health of carers as part of their responsibilities.
- The support provided to carers was to be 'enhanced', in the form of improvements and adaptations to housing, training for carers

(in particular, health and safety around the home issues), and the provision of regular breaks from caring.

The Carers and Disabled Children Act was introduced in the following year, 2000, with the aim of formally strengthening the rights of carers of disabled children to an assessment of their needs. It also gave councils more powers to directly support carers, and in support of this goal it introduced a voucher scheme for carers to have short-term breaks. These new rights for carers were built upon with the introduction of The Carers (Equal Opportunities) Act in 2004. This piece of legislation actually began as a Private Members Bill supported by the carers' lobby group, 'Carers UK', the aim being to enshrine the rights of all carers to be informed of their entitlement to an assessment of their needs, as many carers at the local level had remained unaware of their rights despite the government hype surrounding the introduction of its National Carers strategy. The Bill eventually garnered government support, and received Royal assent in July 2004. The Act placed a duty on councils to consider equality of opportunity for all aspects of a carer's life, including work, study or leisure activities when carrying out a needs assessment. It also sought to promote better joint working between CASSRs and the health service in order to ensure support for carers was delivered in a coherent manner and involved carers in the planning process, as well as providing a specific duty to consider assistance in relation to individual carers. Carers were also for the first time given the opportunity to discuss alternative care services.

Although the needs of carers have finally achieved some prominence in policy development over the past decade, given the narrow way in which social needs are defined in social care, it is difficult to say whether carers themselves now feel better supported and 'recognised' by the statutory agencies. Nevertheless, there is undoubtedly a much broader appreciation of the role of the carer in our society, and the way in which it can be thrust upon any one of us.

THE STATE OF SOCIAL CARE: THE NEED FOR FURTHER REFORM?

Gross current expenditure on personal social services in England in 2006–07 was around £20 billion. Of this expenditure, approximately 25 percent was spent on children and families (spending on providing support for children in care accounted for nearly half of this amount), 43 percent was spent on services for older people, and 23 percent on adults aged 18 to 64 with physical and learning disabilities (NHS Information Centre, 2008).

However, because fees are charged for many council social care services, over £2 billion (mainly from charges for residential and nursing care) were 'clawed-back' in 2005–06. These figures do represent a lower level than in 2001–02, when 20 percent of total spending was recovered from service-users. This reduction reflects the shift in policy set out by the government in *Fairer Charging* (DoH, 2003a), and the moves towards the provision of free nursing care in nursing homes and free rehabilitative services. Nevertheless, it is hard to calculate the total expenditure on the social care element of personal social services spending as there are many sources of funding. But the findings of a review of social care commissioned by the King's Fund (Wanless, 2006), using Department of Health figures for 2004/5, put the gross expenditure at around £8 billion.

During 2006–07, an estimated 1.77 million adult clients received a 'package of community care' provided, purchased or supported by their local CASSR; it should be noted that a client may have had more than one type of service provided (see Figure 10.1). With community-based services (which include day care, meals, home help, respite care, transport and adaptations to the home) provided to 1.52 million of these clients (69 percent of whom were aged 65 or over), and the remaining 350,000 clients received residential or nursing home care (provided by the independent and local authority sectors). A total of 1.9 million needs assessments were carried out in 2006–07; 650,000 were new clients and 1.26 million existing clients (who had their needs reviewed – a process involving a formal reassessment of needs). An estimated 2 million new contacts were made to CASSRs (a figure that has remained unchanged since 2005), with just over 1 million

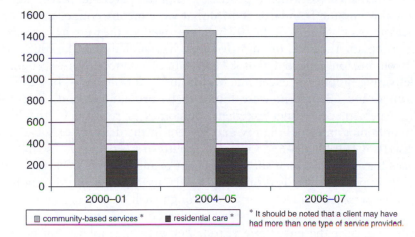

Figure 10.1   Number of clients (in 1000s) receiving community care by service type and age (NHS Information Centre, 2007; DoH, 2001d)

(51 percent) of these adults subsequently receiving an assessment of their needs or the commissioning of an ongoing service. Also in 2006–07, around 393,000 carers received a carers assessment or review, of which 353,000 (90 percent) were taken up. Of those carers assessed, 315,000 (89 percent of total) received a service, of which 56 percent received a 'carer specific' service and 44 percent information only (NHS Information Centre, 2007).

Significantly, whilst both Labour and Conservative governments since 1993 have shared an ideological commitment to shifting the delivery of care from hospitals and care homes to care in the community, the reallocation of expenditure from residential to community services, particularly over the last five years, has been marginal. A report into the state of social care in England, published in January 2008 by the Commission for Social Care Inspection (CSCI), the regulator of care services provided by public, private and voluntary organisations, argued that the reasons for this apparent lack of change were complex, but identified the following factors as significant in the failure to de-institutionalise social care. First, although the number of people financially supported in care homes has fallen since March 2003, the needs of those remaining are greater, and consequently incur greater costs. Second, there has been an increase in the use of residential and nursing beds for rehabilitation, intermediate care and short breaks for carers. Third, at the same time as residential care costs are increasing, patterns of expenditure on community services are changing. People with lower levels of assessed need are increasingly likely to receive fewer or no services (CSCI, 2008: 25).

However, the CSCI reported that it had found, following its inspection and performance assessment processes, that the average percentage of National Minimum Standards (NMS) that were met by council social care services across England in 2006–07 had improved for the fourth consecutive year, although the rate of improvement has stalled (CSCI, 2008: 56). The Commission reported that 83 percent of councils were recognised as delivering 'good' or 'excellent' health and emotional well-being NMS outcomes, and 63 percent were found to be providing 'good' outcomes and 11 percent providing 'excellent' outcomes in relation to the NMS for maintaining personal dignity and respect in the delivery of social care services (CSCI, 2008: 66–69). Overall, the pattern and delivery of social care services for adults has seen some significant changes since 2004, following the shift in policy towards promoting service-user choice and the enabling of greater personal control over care through such measures as increasing direct payments (representing the largest percentage increase of any single service item over the past three years). The greater emphasis on housing with support has also generally been acknowledged as offering people more appropriate and flexible community services.

While people who qualify for social care services are now seeing improvements, the picture can be very different from the perspective of those people who are not eligible for fully-funded council-arranged care. Around half of the total expenditure on personal social care for older people in England comes from private contributions, either from charges and top-ups for those receiving care with council financial support, or from spending on privately purchased care; this figure was estimated to be nearly £5.9 billion in 2005–06 (CSCI, 2008: 108). Table 10.1 shows the estimated numbers of people aged over 65 using both community-based care and care home services. The CSCI estimates that just under 150,000 people were ineligible for council-supported care and were purchasing care privately at the end of 2006. In addition, about a quarter of those in receipt of council-funded community-based care were 'topping-up' their care package through private contributions. In total, of the 750,000 older people using any kind of community-based services, 40 percent of people were paying for some care privately, with most of this spent on residential care (CSCI, 2008: 114). These sums do not include the substantial contribution of resources from private individuals in the form of caring by families and friends.

The 2008 CSCI report strongly criticised the rules that determine which elderly and disabled people in England are entitled to social care. The Commission pointed to the inconsistencies that exist between local authorities when making decisions about who is eligible for help and how much support they should receive. The report found that seven out of ten local authorities currently restrict their services because of restricted budgets for social care to those people whose needs are defined as 'substantial' or 'critical'. The consequence being that there is now a widening gap in social care between social groups, thousands of people who would have got support a few years ago are no longer eligible. The report acknowledges that local councils have had little choice but to seek to find

Table 10.1 The use of social care services by older people, numbers and sources of funding

	Council funded care	Private top-up of council funded care	Private purchase of care	All funding sources
Community-based care	606,000	154,000	145,000 (19% of total)	751,000
Residential care	199,000	70,000	118,000 (37% of total)	317,000
Total	805,000	224,000	263,000	1,068,000

Source: CSCI, 2008

ways to control demand on their finite resources because of a number of factors:

> ... the high costs of care for younger people with complex needs; rising numbers of older people, particularly those who are very elderly, requiring support; and expensive home-based care for people with very intensive needs. Councils, too, have tried to juggle the funding of preventative services at the same time as concentrating resources on people with the greatest needs. (CSCI, 2008: 5–6).

The government has rather belatedly acknowledged these pressures on the social care system, and in October 2007, Alan Johnson, the then Secretary of State for Health, made a statement to the House of Commons which committed the government to a fundamental review of the system within a Green Paper to be published in late 2008. The Comprehensive Spending Review (HM Treasury, 2007), published a few months previously, had already announced an additional increase in social care funding of some £520 million over the next three years. In the interim, the Social Care Minister, Ivan Lewis, ordered a fundamental review of the rules on eligibility in January 2008. In a statement given to BBC Radio, he said the system faced a particular challenge coping with increasing numbers of elderly people developing dementia:

> (T)he health service will in the future have to spend significantly more resources on specialist support for families experiencing dementia: it is the new heart care, the new cancer care, the new stroke care – dementia is one of the great issues we now have to face up to' (BBC On-line, 16 January 2008).

The big question that will posed of this government's review of its social care policy is whether it is prepared to grasp the nettle that is the state provision of non-means tested social care and support as is now provided in Scotland. The government's policy concern with promoting the consumerist choice agenda and a supplier market in health and social care provision would suggest that this is not going to happen in the short to medium term, particularly given the distinct possibility of global economic recession over the next few years.

ACTIVITY

The current government and its successor (whether New Labour is re-elected or replaced by the Conservative Party in office, or some less likely combination) will have to face up to some important decisions over the next five to ten years concerning the future course of social care policy. For the sake of simplicity, this has been reduced to three possible policy options, which are listed below. Think about each possible option in turn and write down in the box below what you think may be the consequences in terms of: (a) funding, (b) equity of provision and (c) personal responsibility, of adopting either of the three courses of action (or inaction).

In order to complete this exercise, think about the models of public policy-making that were outlined in Chapter 3. In particular, whether the development of social care policy over the past decade in particular could be said to be following a 'path-dependency' or clear trajectory, or whether it appears to you to be more characteristic of the 'garbage can' model, in which decisions are made pragmatically in response to pressures and tensions existing at a particular period and context – a useful source of information is a King's Fund Report published in 2008, The Future of Care Funding: Time for a change (available to download for free direct from the King's Fund – www.kingsfund.org.uk.).

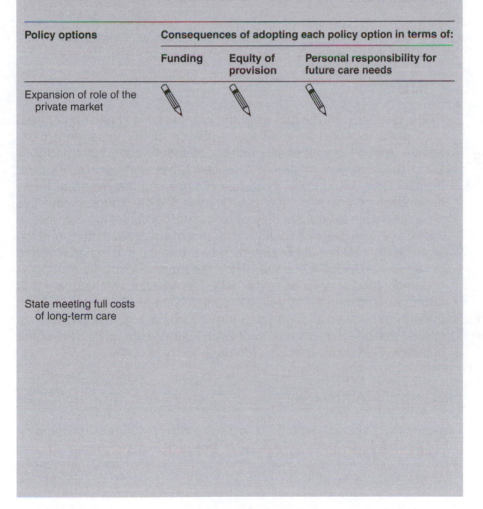

Policy options	Consequences of adopting each policy option in terms of:		
	Funding	Equity of provision	Personal responsibility for future care needs
Expansion of role of the private market			
State meeting full costs of long-term care			

Continued Policy options	Consequences of adopting each policy option in terms of:		
	Funding	Equity of provision	Personal responsibility for future care needs
Status quo – no further reform			

SUMMARY

In this chapter we have looked at the ways in which health and social care policy directed at meeting the needs of the dependent older people and other vulnerable groups has developed spasmodically since the inception of the welfare state over sixty years ago. For the first forty years of the existence of the NHS, the needs of these dependent groups and their carers were largely marginalised: this situation began to improve only with the introduction of the community care framework. Despite continuing issues of under-resourcing and the ongoing distinct lack of collaboration between the two main providers of services – CASSRs and the NHS – the range and quality of support has undoubtedly improved since 1993. The question remains, whether future governments will be willing to continue this level of state provision through general taxation of long-term social care services, given the demographic fact that the ratio of over-75-year-olds to the rest of the population will continue to rise for many years to come.

FURTHER READING

Glendenning, C., Powell, M. and Rummery, K. (eds) (2002) *Partnerships, New Labour and the Governance of Welfare*. Bristol: Policy Press.
Wanless, D. (2006) *Securing Good Care for Older People: Taking a Long-term View*. London: King's Fund.

PART FOUR

LOOKING TO THE FUTURE

11   HEALTH BEYOND POLICY

INTRODUCTION

Health policy in the UK, as we have shown throughout this textbook, is primarily concerned with healthcare provision or more precisely with the clinical management of people who already have ill-health. Public health and preventative health policies, which can be defined as action taken at a societal level in order to protect and promote the health of the whole population, has traditionally held a marginal place in the activity and funding of the NHS. Public health has also been marginalised internationally, as a consequence of the penetration of national economies by global market forces which undermine attempts by national governments to maintain collective responsibility for health and social welfare. At a national level (not confined to the UK) we have seen that healthcare system reforms have focused on cost-containment of medical services and not embraced the need to engage with developing collective public health responses to increasing threats to the global environment and the health of all of us.

The potential to systematically calculate 'risk' (see Key Concept below), in relation to the disease outcomes of certain health behaviours, has become central to an ongoing debate surrounding the changing relationship of governance that pertains between citizens and the state in terms of lifestyles and personal freedom. From being primarily regarded as social and environmental in origin and therefore out of the control of individuals (hence the traditional interventionist role for the state to mitigate what are euphemistically known as the 'externalities' of the capitalist market economy), health risks are increasingly associated with individual 'lifestyle choices' in a consumerist society. The strategy of 'health promotion' as it has been developed and implemented over the past thirty years by both Conservative and New Labour governments, is characterised by an approach that sees the consequences of personal health behaviour as an individual rather than as a state responsibility. This narrow policy focus on attempting to change the behaviour of individuals and 'at-risk' social groups has, with perhaps the exception of smoking, been largely a fruitless activity. Levels of childhood asthma, diabetes, and obesity have soared over the same period of time.

Systematic and persistent social inequalities continue to remain a key characteristic of the social structure of contemporary Britain. Despite sixty years of universal and free healthcare these wider social inequalities are reflected in differential health outcomes between social classes that have grown wider over time. A social gradient of mortality and morbidity rates exists with the highest rates of ill-health and lowest levels of life expectancy found in the unskilled socio-economic classes, and the lowest rates of illness and highest levels of life expectancy found among the most economically and socially privileged social groups. This chapter focuses on the reasons why post-war governments have, until relatively recently, failed to even address these social differences in health outcomes. It then moves on to critically examine the practical commitment of the New Labour government to meeting its stated explicit goal of reducing inequalities in health.

This final section of chapter will explore the attempts to come to terms with the limitations of national policy-making in the face of global environmental processes influencing all our health. Before discussing these policy development issues in detail, it is necessary to engage with the concept of 'risk', a concept which underpins an understanding of the emergent threats to public health.

KEY CONCEPT: HEALTH RISK

The notion of a risk is no longer just associated with personal fate or chance. Many sociologists would argue that the notion of a 'risk', if it is to be utilised at all, has to be understood within the wider social and environmental context in which the hazards and insecurities of modern industrialised societies occur. These hazards are generally now recognised as being in large part

(Continued)

(*Continued*)

inadvertent outcomes of scientific and technological developments. This conceptualisation (known as the 'Risk Society' thesis after the groundbreaking book of the same name written by Ulrich Beck in 1992) sees these risks to health and well-being as having become universal, reflecting the impact of globalisation in all its forms, political, cultural and economic. Risk, conceptualised in this sense, '… is no longer about private fears of the random unknown. It now involves public perception of universal dangerousness and threat' (Culpitt, 1999: 4).

In response to a heightened public perception of these social and environmental threats, attempts have been made to compensate for risks (they cannot be eliminated) both through calculation (risk analysis, also known as the risk assessment approach) and regulatory legislation (improved health and safety, etc.). A key theoretical assumption of this essentially epidemiological approach is the idea that health risk is a phenomenon that can be constructed out of multi-factorial analysis. So, for example, the relative risk of developing heart disease would, within this approach, be based upon a calculation of the mean values associated with certain 'lifestyle' behaviours, such as smoking, diet and exercise, that are drawn from aggregated population data for heart disease incidence. This is a statistical approach that all too often perceives such calculated health risk factors as being realities or causative agents in their own right, often with little acknowledgement of the social and material context of these health behaviours.

Mullard and Spiker (1998) have argued that the risk society is also an atomised or fragmented society lacking social solidarity, where it is individuals rather than society that take the risks. The following example of how this process operates in relation to health behaviour is provided:

> Individuals accept the risk of smoking since they know that smoking is a hazard to their health. Health professionals, having provided the information, argue that they should withdraw treatment from the individual who chooses to continue to smoke. The individual accepts the risk of smoking and therefore also accepts the responsibility for her or his own health. (Mullard and Spiker, 1998: 138)

This discourse of risk is evident in the Department of Health's public health White Paper, '*Saving Lives: Our Healthier Nation*' (DoH, 1999b) from which the following quote is taken:

> The whole question of risks to health, how they are analysed, assessed, communicated and reduced, has come to the fore during the 1990s … (i.e., the controversies associated with food safety and perceived risks of vaccines) … have highlighted the need for a new relationship between government and

(*Continued*)

(*Continued*)

the public in relation to risk … it is the role of the government to provide information about risk. But in most cases it is for the individual to decide whether to take the risk. And there is a balance between risk and personal freedom. (DoH, 1999b: paras 3.19–25)

Dean (1999) would go on to argue that once risk has been attributed to particular health behaviours, the distinction is then drawn within public health policies between 'active citizens', who are perceived as able to manage their own heath risks, and so-called 'at-risk' social groups who become the object of targeted interventions designed to manage these risks. The notion of 'risky behaviour' serving to construct the socially recalcitrant as distinct from the responsible citizen (Turner, 1987; Lupton, 1995).

THE LIMITATIONS OF PUBLIC HEALTH POLICY: HEALTH, BEHAVIOUR AND LIFESTYLE

The strategy of health promotion represents a central element of government public health interventions over the past thirty years. The field of health promotion itself encompasses, along with its more traditional health educational campaigns, community development, personal skills development, the control over the advertising of 'unhealthy' products, and the monitoring and periodic screening of sub-populations. As has been noted; '(T)he encroachment of health promotion into these areas has multiplied the number of sites for preventive action, and given rise to an endless parade of "at risk" populations and "risky situations"' (Petersen, 1997: 195). In other words, health promotion strategies have been primarily concerned with identifying so-called 'problem' or 'at-risk' groups such as adolescent drug-users, pregnant teenagers, smokers, the 'obese', etc. Interventions are directed at persuading these groups to change or control their behaviour or 'lifestyle' so as to reduce the damage they are perceived to be causing to their health through unprotected sex, smoking, unbalanced diet, etc. – The assumption underlying many health promotion campaigns being that it is individual volitional behaviour that constitutes the primary risk to health. Yet, as one group of epidemiologists who are critical of the attempts to calculate actual risk levels for individuals has pointed out, '(E)pidemiological observational studies usually consider several risk exposures, outcomes, as well as subgroups. This results in multiple statistical tests of hypotheses and a high probability of finding associations that are statistically significant but spurious' (Pocock et al., 2004). By way of contrast, sociologists and others would argue that the notion of a 'health risk' cannot be understood outside of the wider context of the emergent 'Risk society' (see the Key Concept above).

As expressed in its first public health White Paper, *Saving Lives: Our Healthier Nation* (DoH, 1999b), the initial position of the New Labour government was to seek to differentiate between the risks associated with individual behaviour and those which are outside the control of individuals. In the case of the former, the responsibility of government is to provide people with the knowledge and information so that they, '... can make informed decisions in managing their everyday life', while in the case of health risks outside of individual control, government will; '... ensure that measures are in place to protect their health' (DoH, 1999b: para 3.16). The White Paper concludes on this point with the assertion that:

> The whole question of risks to health, how they are analysed, assessed, communicated and reduced, has come to the fore during the 1990s ... (controversies associated with food safety and perceived risks of vaccines) ... have highlighted the need for a new relationship between government and the public in relation to risk ... it is the role of the government to provide information about risk. But in most cases it is for the individual to decide whether to take the risk. And there is a balance between risk and personal freedom. (DoH, 1999b: paras 3.19–25)

However, although seeking to avoid 'victim-blaming', this policy perspective is nevertheless underpinned by many of the assumptions of 'rational choice theory' (discussed in detail in Chapter 3). This is a perspective that sees social life as essentially made up of solitary, self-interested individuals who must by force of circumstance make rational choices after weighing all the possible alternatives. It follows, therefore, that every individual should be given the opportunity to manage and take responsibility for the inherent risks in their life. This position is reflected in the rhetoric of neo-liberal governance, which asserts that the proper role of government is to be concerned with the lessening of external health risks, but not the regulation of personal health behaviour (citizens as agents of their own government). Nevertheless, this position also reflects what has been described as 'the conundrum of neo-liberalism'. That is, the government is seeking to reduce its interventionist role in the life of individuals, whilst '... maintaining that the state ought more properly to be involved in dealing with the consequences of a risk society' (Culpitt, 1999: 15).

CASE STUDY – THE CAMPAIGN TO REDUCE LEVELS OF TEENAGE PREGNANCY IN THE UK

The UK has the highest teenage birth rate in Europe and is second only to the USA in a list of the 28 OECD richest developed nations. Early in its first term of office the New Labour government commissioned the newly created (in 1997) Social Exclusion Unit (SEU) to develop a national strategy to cut these high rates of teenage parenthood. The SEU Report was published in June 1999, and set out the following three targets for action:

- To reduce the rate of teenage conceptions, with the specific aim of halving the rate among under-18s by 2010, with an interim reduction of 15 percent by 2004;
- To set a firmly established downward trend in the under 16 conception rate by 2010;
- To increase the participation of teenage parents in education and work, to reduce their risk of long-term social exclusion.

At the same time as this strategy was being developed, the Teenage Pregnancy Unit (TPU) was established within the Department of Health, its role being to link up the work of several government departments to develop shared objectives. The outcome of this work has been the creation of a network of local teenage pregnancy coordinators bringing together the work of social services, education, housing authorities and the 'Sure Start' programme. A national media campaign was launched in 2000 that focused on the themes of taking control of your life choices and personal responsibility (TPU, 2000). This campaign thus combined a moral message with direct interventions in the lives of young women. However, an important impetus for the campaign has been the financial impact that the rise in the teenage pregnancy rate has had on welfare spending, that is, the costs to the state of supporting young, often single, mothers with children knowing that there is only a limited opportunity for these women to support themselves through full-time work. Here there is a rather different moral message being given to young people, that they should be preparing for the world of work and not 'thoughtlessly' having children until they are in a financially secure position.

This example of a health promotion campaign designed to change the sexual behaviour of young people demonstrates the limited scope of the epidemiological risk-focused approach. Teenage pregnancy is problematised (and yet for most of human history, teenage pregnancy has not been seen as a problem at all, but as something that is both normal and desirable) because of what are seen to be the exacerbatory effects of giving birth on the 'social exclusion' of young women. Teenage pregnancy is perceived by policy-makers as primarily a health behavioural problem (i.e., unprotected sex) that predominately affects young women from lower socio-economic groups. These assumptions then justify young working-class women being identified as an 'at-risk' group with all the attendant dangers of stigma and 'victim-blaming'. A selectivised or targeted health promotion initiative is rolled out, and not surprisingly has little impact on teenage pregnancy rates because it does not get to the root of the social reasons why young working-class women choose to become (not 'fall') pregnant. The most recent figures, published by the Office of National statistics for 2005, show that rates for under-18s have been reduced by 11 percent since 1998. However, the rate for girls under 16 had remained static, and as yet there is no 'firmly established downward trend' (ONS, 2007).

THE FAILURE OF HEALTH POLICY: ADDRESSING SOCIAL INEQUALITIES IN HEALTH

Examining health outcomes from a societal rather than individual perspective produces a very different view of the determinants of health. This is not to say that the biological factors (disease pathogens and genetic disorders) identified by medical science are not determinants of the health of individuals, but rather: '… (w)hat really moves the health of whole societies, adding to or subtracting from the sum of total health, may be factors which account for only a very small part of the individual variation in health and so escape detection'(Wilkinson, 1996: 16). Significant differences in mortality and morbidity rates continue to exist between socio-economic groups in most developed countries. This salient fact serves to remind us that health is a social product as much as it is a biological outcome (this model of the social determinants of health is diagrammatically represented in Figure 11.1).

Individual biological development takes place within a social context which structures life chances, so that advantage and disadvantage tend to cluster cross-sectionally and accumulate longitudinally. That is to say that, at any moment in time epidemiologists are able to identify a clear gradient in health outcomes existing between socio-economic classes (see Figure 11.2). These differences then manifest themselves overtime and are represented by differences in life expectancy (see Figure 11.3). The existence of a clear social gradient in the risk of premature death is demonstrated in Figure 11.2. Here, each successive (more disadvantaged) class has a significantly greater mortality than the preceding class (demonstrated by the arrows in the chart). Since 2001, social class mortality data has been collected using the National Statistics Socio-Economic Classification (NS-SEC), in which classes are defined by occupational characteristics such

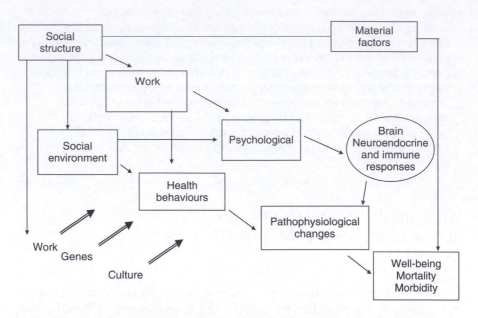

Figure 11.1 Model of social determinants of health (Brunner et al. 1999)

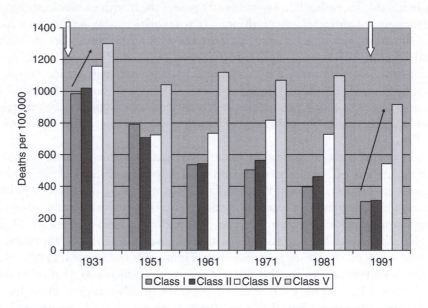

Figure 11.2 Trends in social inequalities in health 1931–1991: Mortality rates per 100,000 men by social class and age, England and Wales

Source: Blane, Bartley and Davey Smith (1997)

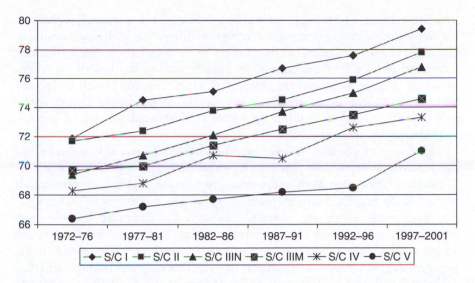

Figure 11.3 Trends in life expectancy at birth by social class, men, England and Wales

Source: ONS Longitudinal Study 1972–2005 (ONS, 2007)

as job control and security of employment, not by income or broader concepts of social position, which was the case for the Registrar-General's Classification (RGC) of social class (utilised in Figure 11.2). Nevertheless, Office of National Statistics (ONS) data for 2001–03 show that men in 'routine' jobs (approximately equivalent to the unskilled, manual Social Class V in the RGC) are 2.8 times more likely to die between the ages of 25 and 64 years than men in higher managerial posts. These figures show little change in health inequalities from the 1991–93 data, when working age men in unskilled manual jobs had 2.9 times the risk of death of those in professional occupations (ONS, 2007).

Life expectancy at birth for a particular social class and time period is an estimate of the number of years a new-born baby would survive were he or she to experience the average age-specific mortality rates of that social class for that time period throughout his or her life. Figure 11.3 demonstrates that people in professional occupations (Social Class I) have the longest expectation of life, followed by managerial and technical occupations (Social Class II), and so on. People in unskilled manual occupations (Social Class V) have the shortest expectation of life.

Inequalities in health outcome in the UK reflect, and are a consequence of, the structured social divisions existing at a particular moment in time. However, in the relationship between health and income, it is the relative income differences that appear to be more important than absolute living standards. The relative income gap that exists in a society, represents for Wilkinson (1996) not only a material difference in living standards but as having psychosocial consequences in terms of the quality of social interrelationships that are ultimately significant for the health outcomes of *all* social groups within that society. That is, a society with wide gaps between rich and poor produces low levels of social cohesion. Social cohesion is defined, following Putnam's (1995) work on social capital, as participation in public life and civic responsibility.

Wilkinson argues that relative income differences strongly influence an individual's perception of place in the social hierarchy – their social status. These perceptions are both internalised, producing negative emotions that impact upon health, and externalised, resulting in anti-social behaviour. The poor become socially marginalised and are therefore less likely to adhere to the norms of that society, resulting in greater levels of crime and personal violence. These are societies where high proportions of the population are in some way excluded from full social participation, and that do not value all its people equally highly (Marmot, 2004). Wilkinson (1996) has argued that a society which has poor health is a society that tolerates or even encourages high income inequality. These outcomes are reflected in Figure 11.4, in which it can be seen that, although the USA has the highest national income (as measured by gross domestic product – GDP), it has a relatively low average life expectancy compared to European countries with lower levels of GDP; in fact it has a life expectancy only slightly higher than that of Cuba. Marmot (2004) uses this type of evidence to draw the

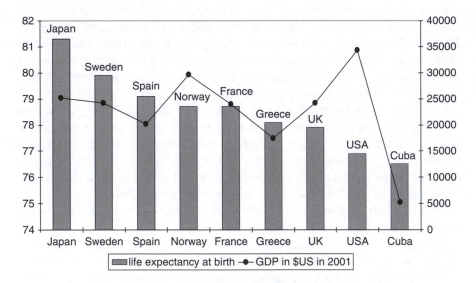

Figure 11.4 Life expectancy and income (OECD, 2005)

conclusion that in the developed world it is not the richest countries that have the best levels of health, but the most egalitarian ones as measured by the gap in income between the rich and poor.

The existence of large differences in mortality and morbidity levels between the rich and the poor were accepted as the norm by policy-makers in pre-war Britain. These differences were seen as an unfortunate consequence of living in a market economy. The post-war political enthusiasm for social justice and change, which led to the establishment of the British Welfare State in the late 1940s, brought with it an expectation that social class differences in health would be narrowed following the provision of free comprehensive medical care for the whole population. However, although the general standard of health improved in the post-war years as measured by average levels of life expectancy, social class differences in health outcome failed to narrow. The official view in the mid-1960s was that the primary cause of these continuing social class differences was behavioural, and that more resources invested in social infrastructure and healthcare provision could not be the solution. This official view ignored social research that was available at the time which challenged the notion that the development of welfare state services had succeeded in eliminating disadvantage in access to health and education services. This so-called 'rediscovery of poverty' in Britain demonstrated that low income continued to be a key factor in social disadvantage.

Health policy from the mid-1970s onward formally incorporated the strategy of health education, with the aim of convincing the population that it was their own health behaviour that required changing (see above). However, this strategy was almost immediately challenged by research then being conducted both in the USA and in Britain. The first 'Whitehall Study' (Marmot et al., 1978) found that differences in health behaviours such as smoking, blood pressure, exercise, and fat intake, were found to account for only a minority of the difference in mortality from coronary heart disease between occupational grades in the Civil Service. The then Labour government responded by setting up a commission to summarise the evidence for social inequalities in health. The Black Report (DHSS, 1979a) as it became known (after its chair, Sir Douglas Black, President of the Royal College of Physicians) was the first modern official report into health inequality in Britain. It closely examined the evidence for an association between social class and health, and demonstrated that mortality and morbidity were not randomly distributed throughout the population. The report identified four possible explanations for this finding. These were: (1) artefact (data errors); (2) social or natural selection, with those with poor health being downwardly mobile; (3) cultural explanations focusing on class differences in health beliefs and behaviour; and (4) material circumstances, in which social differences in income, diet, housing and working environment are the key determinants of inequalities in health. It was the latter explanation of the causes of health inequalities that was accepted by the Black Report and built into its recommendations to government when it was published at the end of 1979. However, the response of the recently elected Conservative government, led by Margaret Thatcher, was to attempt to suppress the findings of the Report by limiting its publication, and to ignore all its recommendations.

Lukes (1974: 2004) theorised power in relation to 'three dimensions' (see Chapter 1): using each of the 'dimensions' as a starting point can offer some of the possible reasons why the Conservative governments of 1979–97 failed to develop any form of policy intervention to address social inequalities in health outcome. In terms of the first 'face' of power, 'formal decision-making', the Lukes model would suggest the Conservative governments did not recognise the depth of the problem and therefore saw no requirement to develop policy to address inequalities in health. In relation to the second dimension, 'non-decision-making', it could be argued that addressing social inequalities was never going to be on the agenda of a Conservative government that was influenced by a neo-liberal ideology which acted to support market forces, even if there were 'fall-outs' in terms of social and health disadvantage for large sections of the population. In relation to the third dimension of power, which examines the manipulation or shaping of the political demands of the population, it could be argued that by the early 1990s, the Conservative government, now in its fourth term and with John Major as Prime Minister, found it difficult to resist the mounting and by now incontrovertible evidence for the widening gap in health between socio-economic classes. So, rather than deny it, the government started talking about 'variations in health' (DoH, 1998a). This approach was one which attempted to persuade us that inequalities were natural and inevitable, and that it was not the job of government to attempt to eradicate them – health was a personal responsibility.

On coming to power in 1997, the New Labour government set about acting upon its long-held commitment to addressing, at least in principle, the issue of social inequalities in health. It commissioned its Chief Medical Officer, Sir Donald Acheson, to produce a report following an independent inquiry into the state of inequalities in health in the UK (very much a follow-up to the Black report which the previous Labour government had commissioned twenty-one years before). The Acheson report (Acheson, 1998) concluded, like the Black report, that material disadvantage was the main determinant of health inequalities. The report made no formal recommendations to government but suggested four forms of state intervention that could have an influence on reducing health inequalities; these were as follows:

- Medical Care interventions – to reduce morbidity to prevent early death;
- Preventative intervention – to change individual health risk;
- Workplace interventions – to improve psychologically stressful conditions;
- Social structural intervention – to reduce social and economic inequalities.

In its first public health White Paper '*Saving Lives: Our Healthier Nation* (DoH, 1999b), the government committed itself to improving the health of the worst-off in society and to narrow the health gap, although no specific targets were set. However, when the *NHS Plan* (DoH, 2000b) was published the following year, an ambitious target was set, which was, ' (t)o reduce inequalities in health outcomes by 10% as measured by infant mortality and life expectancy at birth' (DoH, 2000). This target was underpinned by two more detailed targets, as follows:

- Starting with children under one year old, by 2010 to reduce by at least 10 percent the gap in mortality between manual groups and the population as a whole;
- Starting with Health Authorities, to reduce by at least 10 percent the gap between the quintile of the area with the lowest life expectancy at birth and the population as a whole.

In 2003 the Department of Health published its detailed *Programme of Action for Tackling Health Inequalities* (DoH, 2003b). This set out four areas for intervention (modelled on the Acheson Report recommendations): (1) supporting families to 'break the inter-generational cycle of (ill) health'; (2) to engage communities in identifying local health needs; (3) disease prevention policies; and (4) and not least, 'addressing the underlying determinants of health'. Responsibility for delivering these interventions was to reside with a range of government departments whose actions would be coordinated by the Department of Health. The 'delivery mechanisms' for meeting the Action Programmes' goals included PCTs, local authority social services department, and in particular there was a heavy dependence on the 'Sure Start' local programmes (the community outreach and development initiative).

In assessing New Labour's policy on reducing inequalities in health, the question of 'selectivist' versus 'universalist' provision of public services arises. Although the NHS provides health services on the basis of the principle of equity, as we have seen in Chapter 9, this principle can nevertheless conceal the effects of pre-existing social inequalities, so that the middle classes have actually become the prime beneficiary of the healthcare system. This is the basis for the argument in favour of adopting a more selectivist approach that targets groups and individuals at most social disadvantage. However, in practice, when this approach has been adopted in the context of health promotion interventions (discussed above), it has focused on those groups deemed to have the most 'unhealthy lifestyles'; this has led to charges of government 'victim-blaming'. The selective targeting of people with the highest 'health risks' (usually the lowest socio-economic groups), also ignores the epidemiological evidence of the existence of a social gradient in health outcomes. It might be that those with the lowest socio-economic status have the highest level of health risks, but those with 'average incomes' also have higher levels of morbidity and mortality than those in the top 10 percent of income earners (Mackenbach et al., 2002: 37). This perspective would argue that health policy strategies to reduce inequalities in health should aim at improving the health of the whole population rather than selectively focus, as the Programme of Action largely does, on those who are most disadvantaged.

A status report published by the Department of Health (DoH, 2005c) two years after the instigation of the Programme for Action examined progress in meeting the targets for reductions in health inequalities and makes for sober reading. The report showed that the gap in inequalities in health between Social Class I and Social Class V was actually widening, as measured by infant mortality and life expectancy. There had been some success in reducing the numbers of children in poverty, which had been a New Labour government headline target dating back to 1998, and which reflects the application of 'selectivist' targeted approach discussed above, but overall the trend towards an ever-widening gap in health inequalities continued. The New Labour government could not be directly blamed for the trend, which, as Figure 11.2 shows, dates back to before the Second World War. However, although the Programme for Action demonstrated a political willingness to coordinate government action to meet the targets of reducing health inequalities, this programme has attracted no significant additional funding by the Treasury. Since 2005, efforts by the Department of Health at coordinating action to keep on track to meet the reduction in inequalities, targets appear to have become rather diverted as its focus shifts to delivering its 'supply-led' reforms to the NHS. Since 2005, although the Programme for Action continues in place, there have been few public statements by Ministers of Health on the progress of the programme. The strong impression given is that because there can never be any 'easy-wins' in such an ambitious programme, and that the commitment to reducing inequalities appears to have been de-prioritised by the government.

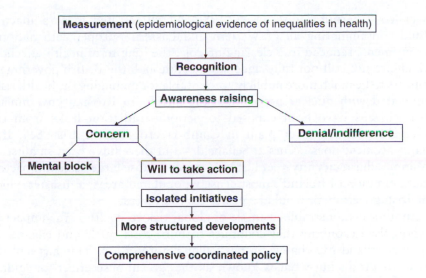

Figure 11.5 **Action spectrum on inequalities in health (Whitehead, 1998)**

Whitehead (1998) has proposed a useful schematic hierarchical 'action spectrum' (see Figure 11.5) in order to illustrate the degree or depth to which health policy could be developed in order to take action on reducing inequalities in health. It is useful to think about these levels in relation in terms of New Labour approach to tackling inequalities. The New Labour government could be said to have reached the level of 'More structured developments' (the previous Conservative government only reached the 'Denial/indifference' level), but efforts to achieve the level of a 'Comprehensive coordinated policy' have been limited following the failure by the Treasury to commit significant public funds towards meeting the goals. It could also be said that there is strong evidence of a failure of will by the government to look beyond the market for solutions to improving wage levels, high quality housing, and reductions in work-related stresses, to identify just three factors complicit in health disadvantage.

WHAT POLICY?: HEALTH AND GLOBAL RISK

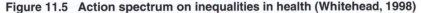

Risks to population health increasingly reflect the process of economic globalisation. In this sense, the managing of health risk is increasingly beyond the control of individual national states and therefore policy-making. Examples of these global risks to health are manifest.

In the case of one of the more obvious examples, the impact of generating electricity by means of nuclear reactors, the most chilling episode was the so-called 'Chernobyl disaster' of 1986, which resulted in a radioactive cloud contaminating all of Western and Eastern Europe, with national governments reduced to a clearing-up role, the long-term health effects of which are not still not fully understood. Although the British government appears to be much more publicly accountable for managing the health risks associated with nuclear power than the Soviet-era Russian government, Irish citizens have been exposed to periodic radiation leaks from the Sellafield nuclear power plant in Cumbria crossing the Irish Sea. If a major accident does occurs at Sellafield – and there have been small scale examples during its fifty-year history – it could cause large-scale radioactive contamination of Ireland's most densely populated areas, a disaster which the Irish government would be powerless to prevent.

Another demonstrable example of global risk to health is the impact of a globalised economy that continues to burn fossil fuels and engages in significant land-use change, in particular deforestation. This has had the effect of producing what is known as the 'greenhouse effect' or 'global warming'. Naturally occurring greenhouse gases have a mean warming effect without which Earth would be uninhabitable, the issue is how the strength of the greenhouse effect changes when human activity increases the atmospheric concentrations of some greenhouse gases such as carbon dioxide and methane in particular. The Intergovernmental Panel on Climate Change (IPCC) has concluded that:

> ... most of the observed increase in globally averaged temperatures since the mid-twentieth century is very likely due to the observed increase in anthropogenic (processes, objects, or materials are those that are derived from human activities, as opposed to those occurring in natural environments without human influences) greenhouse gas concentrations. (IPCC, 2007)

These global effects are clearly beyond the control of any single national government and any reduction in carbon emission policies they may pursue. This is why only an international policy agreement such as that achieved at Kyoto in 1997 has any possibility at all of success. As of 2007, 36 developed countries have agreed to the protocol and have committed themselves to reducing greenhouse gas emissions to the levels specified for each of them in the treaty. One hundred and thirty-seven developing countries have also ratified the protocol, but have no obligation beyond monitoring and reporting emissions.

Other global health risks follow from the greater mobility of populations, in large part resulting from population migration and the development of global air travel. In its wake have come the threats to public health posed by the spread of diseases such as the avian flu pandemic, for example, which was previously confined to a fixed geographical area. Other examples of global disease spread would include HIV/AIDS. Significantly though, the World Health Organisation has predicted that 50 percent more people will die of tobacco-related disease globally than of HIV/AIDS in 2015, reflecting the power of the tobacco industry and its effective worldwide advertising. These examples of global threats to health (and there are countless more), indicate that, increasingly, national governments, if they wish to protect the health of their populations, will need to think about health policy at an international level, coordinated through organisations such as the WHO and the EU. Therefore the key question for governments in the future is whether they will be willing to forgo their policy-making sovereignty for the health of all ?

FURTHER READING

Marmot, M. (2004) *Status Syndrome*. London: Bloomsbury.

Intergovernmental Panel on Climate Change (2007) *Climate Change 2007: The Physical Science Basis. Contribution of Working Group I to the Fourth Assessment Report of the Intergovernmental Panel on Climate Change.* Available at: http://ipcc-wg1.ucar.edu/wg1/Report

NOTES

CHAPTER 6

1 The ratio of the economically dependent part of the population, to the productive part. The economically dependent parts of the population are those who are either too young or too old to work; generally assumed to be those aged below 15 years, or above 64, divided by the number of individuals aged 15 to 64 in the labour force.

2 Healthy life expectancy, or health-adjusted life expectancy (HALE), summarises the number of years to be lived in what might be termed 'full health'. To calculate HALE, the WHO weights the years of ill-health according to severity and subtracts them from overall life expectancy to give the equivalent years of healthy life.

CHAPTER 8

1 The quality adjusted life year (QALY) is a measure of the expected health gain (extending life expectancy or improving the quality of life or both) from a therapeutic intervention or treatment. QALYs are the primary measure of cost-effectiveness used by NICE in its system of medical technology appraisal system. The frequently voiced critique of QALYs as a quality of life measure, is that they prioritise physical functionality (assessed by means of a disability scale), over the social costs (both material and emotional) associated with the experience of living with a chronic illness.

2 The Risk-Sharing Scheme, unlike any other guidance on the cost-effectiveness of medical technology in England and Wales, for the first time established a cost-effectiveness threshold for disease modifying treatments in multiple sclerosis of £36,000 per QALY.

CHAPTER 10

1 The Department of Health define 'social care' as, '(t)he wide range of services designed to support people to maintain their independence, enable them to play a fuller part in society, protect them in vulnerable situations and manage complex relationships'. These social care services are to be distinguished from 'community services', which are defined as, '(t)he full range of services provided outside hospitals by nurses and other health professionals; for example physiotherapists, chiropodists and others (DoH, 2006c).

REFERENCES

Abel-Smith, B. and Townsend, P. (1966) *The Poor and the Poorest*. London Bell.

Acheson Report (1998) *Independent Inquiry into Inequalities in Health*. London: Stationery Office.

Adams, J. and Schmuecker, K. (eds) (2006) *Devolution in Practice 2006*. London: Institute of Public Policy Research (IPPR).

Appleby, J. and Harrison, A. (2006) *Spending on Health: How Much is Enough?* London: Kings Fund.

Archer, M. (1998) 'Social theory and the analysis of society', in May, T. and Williams, M. (eds). *Knowing the Social World*. Buckingham: Open University Press. pp. 69–85.

Baggott, R. (2004) *Health and Health Care in Britain* (3rd edn). Basingstoke: Palgrave MacMillan.

Beck, U. (1992) *Risk Society: Towards a New Modernity*. London: Sage.

Bell, D. (1960) *The End of Ideology*. New York: Free Press.

Berg, J.S., Dischler, J., Wagner, D.J., Raja, J.J. and Palmer-Shevlin, N. (1993) Medication complaince: a healthcare problem. *Annals of Pharmacotherapy* 27(9): 1–24.

Bevan, G. (2006) 'Setting targets for health care performance: Lessons from a case study of the English NHS', *National Institute Economic Review*, 197: 67–79.

Bevan, G. and Hood, C. (2006) 'Have targets improved performance in the English NHS?', *British Medical Journal*, 332: 419–22.

Blair, T. (2003) *Fabian Society Annual Lecture – Progress and Justice in the 21st Century*. London: Fabian Society.

Blank, R. and Burau, V. (2004) *Comparative Health Policy*. Basingstoke: Palgrave Macmillan.

Bradshaw, J. R. (1972) 'The taxonomy of social need', in McLachlan, G. (ed). *Problems and Progress in Medical Care*. Oxford: Oxford University Press.

Braybrooke, D. and Lindblom, C. (1963) *A Strategy of Decision*. New York: Free Press.

Brittain, S. (1977) *The Economic Consequences of Democracy*. London: Temple Smith.

Brunner, E., Marmot, M. and Wilkinson, R. (1999) *Social Determinants of Health*. Oxford: Oxford University Press.

Busse, R. Saltman, R. and Dubois, H. (2004) 'Organization and financing of social insurance systems; current status and recent policy developments', in Saltman, R., Busse, R. Figueras, J. (eds). *Social Health Insurance Systems in Western Europe*. Maidenhead: Open University Press. pp. 33–80.

Cabinet Office (1999) *Modernising Government*. Cmnd 4310. London: Stationery Office.

Cabinet Office Strategic Policy Making Team (1999) *Professional Policy Making for the Twenty-First Century* – www.policyhub.gov.uk/docs/prof policymaking.pdf

Chang, L. (2007) 'The NHS performance assessment framework as a balanced scorecard approach: limitations and implications', *International Journal of Public Sector Management*, 20(2): 101–117.

Clarke, J. (1998) 'Thriving on Chaos? Managerialisation and Social Welfare', in Carter, J. (ed). *Postmodernity and the Fragmentation of Welfare*. London: Routledge. pp. 171–187.

Clarke, J. (2004) *Changing Welfare, Changing States: New directions in social policy*. London: Sage.

Clarke, J. and Newman, J. (1997) *The Managerial State*. London: Sage.

Clarke, J. and Newman, J. (2006) The People's choice? citizens, consumers and public services. Paper for International workshop: *Citizenship and Consumption: Agency, Norms, Mediations and Spaces*. Cambridge: Kings College, Cambridge.

Clasen, J. (2004) 'Defining comparative social policy', in Kennet, P. (ed). *A Handbook of Comparative Social Policy*. Cheltenham: Edward Elgar. pp. 91–102.

Clegg, S. (1994) 'Max Weber and the contemporary sociology of organisations', in Ray, L. and Reed, M. (eds). *Organizing Modernity: New Weberian Perspectives on Work, Organization and Society*. London: Routledge. pp. 46–80.

Coffey, A. (2004) *Reconceptualizing Social Policy*. Maidenhead: Open University Press.

Commission for Social Care Inspection (2008) *The State of Social Care in England 2006–07*. London: CSCI.

Cooper, R. and Burrell, G. (1989) 'Modernism, postmodernism and organisational analysis: An introduction', *Organisational Studies*, 9(1): 91–112.

Crinson, I. (2004) 'The Politics of Regulation Within the 'Modernised' NHS: the case of beta interferon and the 'cost-effective' treatment of multiple sclerosis', *Critical Social Policy*, 24(1): 30–49.

Crinson, I. (2008) 'The Health Professions', in Scambler, G. (ed). *Sociology as Applied to Medicine* (6th edn). London: Elsevier. pp. 252–264.

Crinson, I., Shaw, A., Durrant, R., de Lusignan, S. and Williams, B. (2007) 'Coronary Heart Disease and the Management of Risk: Patient Perspectives of outcomes associated with the clinical implementation of the National Service Framework Targets', *Health, Risk and Society*, 9(4): 1–15.

Culpitt, I. (1999) *Social Policy and Risk*. London: Sage.

Cutler, T. and Waine, B. (1997) *Managing the Welfare State: The Politics of Public Sector Management*. Oxford: Berg.

Dahl, R. A. (1957) *The Concept of Power*. New York: Bobbs-Merrill.

Davies, C. (2003) 'Introduction: a New Workforce in the Making?', in Davies, C. (ed). *The Future Health Workforce*. Basingstoke: Palgrave. pp. 1–13.

Davies, H. (2002) 'Understanding organizational culture in reforming the NHS', *Journal of the Royal Society of Medicine*, 95: 140–142.

Dean, M. (1999) *Governmentality, Power and Rule in Modern Society*. London: Sage.

Department of Health and Social Security (1979a) *Inequalities in Health: Report of a Research Working Group Chaired by Sir Douglas Black*. London: HMSO.

Department of Health and Social Security (1979b) *Patients First : Consultative Paper on the Structure and Management of the NHS in England and Wales*. London: HMSO.

Department of Health and Social Security (1983) *NHS Management Inquiry* (The Griffiths Management Report). London: DHSS.

Department of Health (1989a) *Working for Patients*. Cmnd 555. London: HMSO.

Department of Health (1989b) *Caring for People: Community Care in the Next Decade and Beyond*. Cmnd 849. London: HMSO.

Department of Health (1992) *The Health of the Nation*. Cm 1986. London: HMSO.

Department of Health (1997a) *The New NHS: Modern, Dependable*. Cm 3807. London: HMSO.

Department of Health (1997b) *Community Care Statistics: Day and Domiciliary Personal Social Services for Adults, England 1996*. London: DoH.

Department of Health (1998a) *Our Healthier Nation*. Cm 3852. London: Stationery Office.

Department of Health (1998b) *A First Class Service*. London: DoH.

Department of Health (1999a) *Departmental Report 1999*. London: DoH.

Department of Health (1999b) *Saving Lives: Our Healthier Nation*. London: Stationery Office.

Department of Health (2000a) *A Health Service of All the Talents: Developing the NHS Workforce: A Framework for Lifelong Learning for the NHS*. London: DoH.

Department of Health (2000b) *The NHS Plan: A Plan for Investment, A Plan for Reform*. Cmnd 4818. London: The Stationery Office.

Department of Health (2000c) *National Service Framework for Coronary Heart Disease*. London: DoH.

Department of Health (2001a) *Departmental Report 2001*. London: DoH.

Department of Health (2001b) *NHS Performance Ratings Acute Trusts 2000/01*. London: DoH.

Department of Health (2001c) *National Service Framework for Older People in England and Wales*. London: DoH.

Department of Health (2001d) *Community Care Statistics 2003–43: Referrals, Assessments and Packages of Care for Adults*. London: DoH.

Department of Health (2002) *Delivering the NHS Plan: Next Steps on Investment, Next Steps on Reform*. London: Stationery Office.

Department of Health (2003a) *Fairer Charging Policies for Home Care and Other Non-residential Social Services*. London: Department of Health.

Department of Health (2003b) *Tackling Health Inequalities: A Programme for Action*. London: DoH.

Department of Health (2004a) *Departmental Report 2004*. London: DoH.

Department of Health (2004b) *Agenda for Change*. London: DoH.

Department of Health (2004c) *The NHS Improvement Plan: Putting People at the Heart of Public Service*. Cm 6268. London: The Stationery Office.

Department of Health (2004d) *General Medical Services Statement of Financial Entitlements (SFE) 2004/5*. London: DoH.

Department of Health (2005a) *Creating a Patient-led NHS – Delivering the NHS Improvement Plan*. London: DoH.

Department of Health (2005b) *Health Reform in England: Update and Next Steps*. London: DoH.

Department of Health (2005c) *Tackling Health Inequalities: Status Report on the Programme for Action*. London: DoH.

Department of Health (2006a) *Departmental Report 2006*. London: DoH.

Department of Health (2006b) *The NHS in England: The Operating Framework for 2006/07*. London: Department of Health.

Department of Health (2006c) *Our Health, Our Care, Our Say: A New Direction for Community Services*. London: The Stationery Office.

Department of Health (2007a) *Trust, Assurance and Safety – The Regulation of Health Professionals in the 21st Century*. Cm 7013. London: The Stationery Office.

Department of Health (2007b) *The NHS in England: The Operating Framework for 2007/08 Choice at Referral – Guidance Framework for 2006/07*. London: DoH.

Department of Health (2007c) *Free Choice in Elective Care: Equality Impact Assessment*. London: DoH.

Department of Health (2007d) *Our NHS Our future: NHS Next Stage Review – Interim Report*. London: DoH.

Department of Health (2007e) *Social Care PFI initiative* (Gateway ref 8451). www.dh.gov.uk/en/Procurementandproposals/Publicprivatepartnership/Privatefinanceinitiative/SocialCarePFIInitiative/index.htm – accessed February 2008.

Department of Health, Social Services, and Public Safety (2008) *Proposals for Health and Social Care Reform*. Belfast: DHSSPS.

Dixon, S. (2008) *Report on the National Patient Choice Survey – September 2007 England*. London: DoH.

Dowell, J. and Hudson, H. (1997) 'A qualitative study of medication-taking behaviour in primary care', *Family Practice*, 14: 369–375.

Downs, A. (1957) *An Economic Theory of Democracy*. New York: Harper and Row.

Dowswell, G., Harrison, S. and Wright, J. (2002) 'The early days of primary care groups: general practitioners' perceptions', *Health and Social Care in the Community*, 10: 46–54.

Doyal, L. (1976) *The Political Economy of Health*. London: Pluto.

Dunleavy, P. (1986) 'Explaining the privatization boom: public choice versus radical approaches', *Public Administration*, 64(1): 13–34.

Dunleavy, P. (1991) *Democracy, Bureaucracy and Public Choice*. Hemel Hempstead: Harvester Wheatsheaf.

Duran, A., Sheiman, I., Schneider, M. and Øvretveit, J. (2005) 'Purchasers, providers and contracts', in Figueras, J., Robinson, R. and Jakubowski, E. (eds). *Purchasing to Improve Health Systems Performance*. Maidenhead: Open University Press. pp. 187–214.

Eagleton, T. (1991) *Ideology*. London: Verso.

Eldridge, J. (1994) 'Work and authority: some Weberian perspectives', in Ray, L. and Reed, M. (eds). *Organizing Modernity: New Weberian Perspectives on Work, Organization and Society*. London: Routledge. pp. 81–97.

Elmore, R. (1982) 'Backward mapping: Implementation research and policy decision', in Williams, W. (ed). *Studying Implementation: Methodological and Administrative Issues*. Chatam, NJ: Chatham House.

Elston, M-A. (1991) 'The politics of professional power: medicine in a changing health service', in Gabe, J., Calnan, M. and Bury, M. (eds). *The Sociology of the Health Service*. London: Routledge. pp. 58–88.

Evans, P. Rueschemeyer, D. and Skocpol, T. (eds) (1985) *Bringing the State Back in*. Cambridge: Cambridge University Press.

Exworthy, M., Wilkinson, E., McColl, A., Moore, M., Roderick, P., Smith, H. and Gabbay, J. (2003) 'The role of performance indicators in changing the autonomy of the general practice profession in the U.K', *Social Science and Medicine*, 56: 1493–1504.

Farrington-Douglas, J. and Allen, J. (2005) *Equitable Choices for Health*. London: IPPR.

Figueras, J., Saltman, R., Busse, R. and Dubois, H. (2004) 'Patterns and performance in social health insurance systems', in Saltman, R., Busse, R. and Figueras, J. (eds). *Social Health Insurance Systems in Western Europe*. Maidenhead: Open University Press. pp. 81–140.

Flinders, M. (2006) 'Public/Private: The Boundaries of the State', in Hay, C., Lister, M. and Marsh, D. (eds). *The State: Theories and Issues*. Basingstoke: Palgrave Macmillan. pp. 223–246.

Foucault, M. (1979a) *The History of Sexuality: Volume 1*. Harmondsworth: Penguin Books.

Foucault, M. (1979b) Governmentality, *Ideology and Consciousness*. no 6: 5–26.

Foucault, M. (1980) *Power/knowledge: selected interviews*. London: Harvester Wheatsheaf.

Fraser, D. (1973) *The Evolution of the British Welfare State*. Basingstoke: Macmillan Press.

Freeman, R. (2000a) *The Politics of Health in Europe*. Manchester: Manchester University Press.

Freeman, R. (2000b) *Health Policy and the Problem of Learning*, unpublished working paper available at University of Edinburgh Politics website (www.pol.ed.ac.uk).

Friedman, M. (1962) *Capitalism and Freedom*. Chicago: University of Chicago Press.

Friedson, E. (1970) *The Profession of Medicine*. London: University of Chicago Press.

Friedson, E. (1994) *Professionalism Reborn*. Cambridge: Polity Press.

Friedson, E. (2001) *Professionalism: The Third Logic*. Cambridge: Policy Press.

Fukuyama, F. (1992) *The End of History and the Last of Man*. New York: Free Press.

Gabe, J., Calnan, M. and Bury, M. (eds) (1991) *The Sociology of the Health Service*. London: Routledge.

Gaffney, D., Pollack, A., Price, D. and Shaoul, J. (1999) 'NHS capital expenditure and the private finance initiative – expansion or contraction?', *British Medical Journal*, 319(7201): 48.

Garton Ash, T. (2007) 'Europe's true stories', *Prospect*, Issue 131, Feb 2007: 36–41.

Giddens, A. (1976) *New Rules of Sociological Method*. London: Hutchinson.

Glendinning, C. and Means, R. (2004) 'Rearranging the deckchairs on the Titanic of long-term care – is organisational integration the answer?', *Critical Social Policy*, 24(4): 435–457.

Goddard, M. and Smith, P. (2001) 'Equity of access to health care services', *Social Science and Medicine*, 53: 1149–1162.

Gough, I. (1979) *The Political Economy of the Welfare State*. Basingstoke: Macmillan.

Gramsci, A. (1971) in Hoare, Q. and Nowell-Smith, G. (eds). *Selections from Prison Notebooks*. London: Lawrence and Wishart.

Gray, A. (2004) 'Governing medicine: An introduction', in Gray, A. and Harrison, S. (eds). *Governing Medicine; Theory and Practice*. Maidenhead: Open University Press. pp. 5–20.

Greener, I. (2001) '"The ghost of health services past" revisited: Comparing British health policy of the 1950s with the 1980s and 1990s', *International Journal of Health services*, 31(3): 635–646.

Griffiths, R. (1988) *Community Care: An Agenda for Action*. A Report to the Secretary of State for Social Services. London: HMSO.

Hadley, R. and Clough, R. (1997) *Care in Chaos: Frustration and Challenge in Community Care*. London: Cassell.

Ham, C. (1992) *Health Policy in Britain* (2nd edn). Basingstoke: Macmillan.

Hay, C. (2006) '(What's Marxist about) Marxist State Theory', in Hay, C., Lister, M. and Marsh, D. (eds). *The State: Theories and Issues*. Basingstoke: Palgrave Macmillan. pp. 59–78.

Haug, M. and Lavin, B. (1983) *Consumerism in Medicine: Challenging Physician Authority*. Beverley Hills: Sage.

Hayek, F. (1982) *Law, Legislation and Liberty*. 3 vols. London: Routledge and Kegan Paul.

Healthcare Commission (2005) *Performance Rating*. London: Stationery Office.

Healy, P. (1993) 'Arrangements for care', *Nursing Times*, 89(3): 26–29.

Held, D. (ed) (1983) *States and Societies*. Oxford: Blackwell.

Hernes, H. M. (1988) 'Scandanavian citizenship', *Acta Sociologica*, 31(3): 199–215.

Higgins, J. (1986) 'Comparative social policy', *The Quarterly Journal of Social Affairs*, 2(3): 221–242.

Hill, M. (1997) *The Policy process in the Modern State* (3rd edn). London: Prentice Hall.

Hill, M. (2004) *The Public Policy Process* (4th edn). Harlow: Pearson Longman.

HM Treasury (2004) *Comprehensive Spending Review 2004*. London: HM Treasury.

HM Treasury (2006) *Public Expenditure Statistical Analysis 2006*. www.hm-treasury.gov.uk/documents/public_spending_and_services – accessed May 2006.

HM Treasury (2007) *Comprehensive Spending Review 2007*. London: HM Treasury.

Hogwood, B. and Gunn, L. (1984) *Policy Analysis for the Real World*. Oxford: Oxford University Press.

Hood, C. (1976) *The Limits of Administration*. London: Wiley.

Hood, C. (1991) 'A public management for all seasons', *Public Administration*, 69: 3–19.

Hood, C. and Peters, G. (2004) 'The middle aging of the New Public Management: into the age of paradox?', *Journal of Public Administration Research and Theory*, 14(3): 267–282.

Hood, C. and Scott, C. (2000) *Regulating Government in a 'Managerial' Age: Towards a Cross-National Perspective*. London: Centre for Analysis of Risk and Regulation, LSE.

Hood, C., Scott, C., James, O., Jones, G. and Travers, T. (1999) *Regulation inside Government*. Oxford: Oxford University Press.

House of Commons Health Select Committee (2007) *The Electronic Patient Record – Sixth Report of Session 2006–07. HC 4224*. London: The Stationery Office.

Hudson, B. and Henwood, M. (2002) 'The NHS and Social Care: The Final Countdown?', *Policy and Politics*, 30(2): 152–166.

Intergovernmental Panel on Climate Change (2007) *Climate Change 2007:*

The Physical Science Basis. Contribution of Working Group I to the Fourth Assessment Report of the Intergovernmental Panel on Climate Change. http://ipcc-wg1.ucar.edu/wg1/Report – accessed December 2007.

Jessop, B. (1984) *The Capitalist State.* Oxford: Basil Blackwell.

Jessop, B. (1990) *State Theory: Putting Capitalist States in their Place.* Cambridge: Polity Press.

Jessop, B. (1994) 'The transition to post-Fordism and the Schumpeterian workfare state', in Burrows, R. and Loader, B. (eds). *Towards a Post-Fordist Welfare State?* London: Routledge.

Jessop, B. (1999) Narrating the Future of the National Economy and the National State? Remarks on Remapping Regulation and Reinventing Governance, published by Department of Sociology, Lancaster University, Lancaster, at http://www.comp.lancs.ac.uk/sociology/papers/Jessop-Narrating-the-Future.pdf

Jessop, B. (2002) *The Future of the Capitalist State.* Cambridge: Polity Press.

Jessop, B. (2000a) 'From the KWNS to the SWPR', in Lewis, G., Gerwirtz, S. and Clarke, J. (eds). (2000) *Rethinking Social Policy.* London: Sage.

Jessop, B. (2000b) 'Institutional (Re)Turns and the Strategic-Relational Approach', published by the Department of Sociology, Lancaster University, Lancaster, at http://www.comp.lancs.ac.uk/sociology/papers/Jessop-institutional-(Re)turns.pdf

Johnson, T. (1982) 'The state and the professions: peculiarities of the British', in Giddens, A. and MacKenzie (eds). *Social Class and the Division of Labour.* Cambridge: Cambridge University Press.

Jones, C. and Munro, R. (eds) (2005) *Contemporary Organisation Theory.* Oxford: Blackwell Publishing/ The Sociological Review.

Kantola, J. (2006) 'Feminism', in Hay, C., Lister, M. and Marsh, D. (eds). *The State: Theories and Issues.* Basingstoke: Palgrave Macmillan. pp. 118–134.

Kennedy, I. (2001) *The Report of the Bristol Royal Infirmary Inquiry.* London: The Stationery Office.

Kings Fund Report (2006) *Designing the 'new' NHS: Ideas to Make a Supplier Market in Health Care Work.* London: Kings Fund.

Kings Fund Report (2008) *The Future of Care Funding: Time for a Change.* London: Kings Fund.

Klein, R. (1990) 'The state and the profession: the politics of the double bed', *British Medical Journal*, 301: 700–702.

Klein, R. (1995) *The New Politics of the NHS* (3rd edn). London: Longman.

Klein, R. (2001) *The New Politics of the NHS* (4th edn). Harlow: Pearson.

Klein, R. (2004) 'Britain's National Health Service Revisited', *New England Journal of Medicine*, 350(9): 937–942.

Kuhlmann, E. (2006) *Modernising Health Care: Reinventing Professions, the State and the Public.* Cambridge: Policy Press.

Lane, J. E. (2000) *The Public Sector: Concepts, Models and Approaches* (3rd edn). London: Sage.

Langan, M. (1998) 'Rationing Health Care', in Langan, M. (ed). *Welfare: Needs, Rights and Risks*. London: Routledge. pp. 35–80.

Larrain, J. (1979) *The Concept of Ideology*. London: Hutchinson.

Larrain, J. (1983) *Marxism and Ideology*. Basingstoke: Macmillan.

Larson, M. (1977) *The Rise of Professionalism: A Sociological Analysis*. London: University of California Press.

Le Grand, J., Mays, N. and Dixon, J. (1998) 'The Reforms: Success or failure or neither?', in Le Grand, J., Mays, N. and Mulligan, J. (eds). *Learning from the NHS Internal Market: A Review of Evidence*. London: King's Fund. pp. 117–143.

Le Grand, J., Dixon, A., Henderson, J., Murray, R. and Poteliakhoff, E. (2003) *Is the NHS equitable? A Review of the Evidence*. LSE Health and Social Care Discussion Paper No 11. London: London School of Economics and Political Science.

Lewis, D., Robinson, J. and Wilkinson, E. (2003) 'Factors involved in deciding to start preventative treatment : qualitative study of clinicians and lay people's attitudes', *British Medical Journal*, 327: 841–847.

Lindblom, C. (1965) *The Intelligence of Democracy*. New York: Free Press.

Lindblom, C. (1977) *Politics and Markets*. New York: Basic Books.

Local Government Management Board (1997) *Community Care Trends: 1997 Report*. London: Local Government Management Board.

Lowe, R. (1993) *The Welfare State in Britain since 1945*. Basingstoke: Macmillan.

Lukes, S. (1974) *Power: A Radical View*. Basingstoke: Macmillan.

Lukes, S. (2004) *Power: A Radical View* (2nd edn). London: Palgrave.

Lupton, D. (1995) *The Imperative of Health: Public Health and the Regulated Body*. London: Sage.

Macdonald, K. (1995) *The Sociology of the Professions*. London: Sage.

Mackenbach, J., Bakker. M., Sihto, M. and Diderichsen, F. (2002) 'Strategies to reduce socioeconomic inequalities in health', in Mackenbach, J. and Bakker, M. (eds). *Reducing Inequalities in Health: A European Perspective*. London: Routledge.

Mahoney, J. (2000) 'Path dependence in historical sociology', *Theory and Society*, 29: 507–548.

Mannion, R., Davies, H. and Marshall, M. (2005) 'Impact of star performance ratings in English acute hospital trusts', *Journal of Health Services Research and Policy*, 10(1): 18–24.

Maor, M. (1999) 'The paradox of managerialism', *Public administration Review*, 59(1): 5–18.

March, J. and Olsen, J. (eds) (1976) *Ambiguity and Choice in Organisations*. Oslo: Universitetsforlaget.

Marmot, M. Rose, G., Shipley, M., and Hamilton, P. (1978) 'Employment grade and coronary heart disease in British civil servants', *Journal of Epidemiology and Community Health*, 32: 244–249.

Marmot, M. (2004) *Status Syndrome*. London: Bloomsbury.

Marshall, T. H. (1950) *Citizenship and Social Class and other Essays.* Cambridge: Cambridge University Press.

Marshall, M. (2002) *The Publication of Performance Data in the National Health Service.* London: NHS.

Martin, B. (1998) 'Knowledge, identity and the middle class: from collective to individualised class formation?', *Sociological Review*, 46: 653–687.

McKinlay, J. and Arches, J. (1985) 'Towards the proletarianization of physicians', *International Journal of Health Services*, 18: 191–205.

Means, R., Richards, S. and Smith, R. (2002) *From Community Care to Market Care? The Development of Welfare Services for Older People.* Bristol: Policy Press.

Merrison Commission (1979) *Report of the Royal Commission on the NHS.* Cmnd 7615. London: HMSO.

Milewa, T. and Barry, C. (2005) 'Health Policy and the Politics of Evidence', *Social Policy & Administration*, 39(5): 498–512.

Mills, C. W. (1956) *The Power Elite.* Oxford: Oxford University Press.

Ministry of Health (1957) *Local Authority Services for the Chronic Sick and Infirm Circular 14/57.* London: Ministry of Health.

Mishra, R. (1993) 'Social policy in the postmodern world', in Jones, C. (ed). *New Perspectives on the Welfare State in Europe.* Routledge: London.

Mohan, J. (1996) 'Accounts of the NHS reforms: macro-, meso- and micro-level perspectives', *Sociology of Health and Illness*, 18(5): 675–698.

Moran, M. (2004) 'Governing Doctors in the British Regulatory State', in Gray, A. and Harrison, S. (eds). *Governing Medicine; Theory and Practice.* Maidenhead: Open University Press. pp. 27–36.

Mosca, G. (1939) *The Ruling Class.* New York: McGraw Hill.

Mueller, D. (1979) *Public Choice.* Cambridge: Cambridge University Press.

Mueller, D. (1989) *Public Choice II.* Cambridge: Cambridge University Press.

Mullard, M. and Spiker, P. (1998) *Social Policy in a Changing World.* London: Routledge.

National Assembly for Wales (2001) *Improving Health in Wales: A Plan for the NHS with its Partners.* Cardiff: National Assembly for Wales.

New, B. (1996) 'The rationing agenda in the NHS', *British Medical Journal*, 312: 1593–1601.

Newman, J. (2001) *Modernising Governance.* London: Sage.

NHS Executive (1999) *HSC 1999/176 – NICE: initial work programme.* London: DoH.

NHS Information Centre (2007) *Community Care Statistics 2006–07: Referrals, Assessments and Packages of Care for Adults, England: National Summary.* London: NHS.

NHS Information Centre (2008) *Personal Social Services Expenditure and Unit Costs: England 2006/07.* London: NHS.

NICE (2000a) *Appraisal of the use of beta interferons in the treatment of multiple sclerosis: Decision of the Appeal Panel 22/23 September 2000.* London: DoH.

NICE (2000b) *Press Release 2000/052 – NICE to commission further research on MS drugs.*

NICE (2001) *Press Release 2001/034 - Discussions between the Department of health and manufacturers of beta interferon.*

NICE (2002a) *Technology Appraisal guidance No 32 – Beta interferon and glatiramer acetate for the treatment of multiple sclerosis.* London: DoH.

NICE (2002b) *Press Release 2002/007 – NICE issues guidance on drugs for multiple sclerosis.*

Nordhaus, W. (1975) 'The political business cycle', *Review of Economic Studies,* Vol. 42: 169–190.

NPfIT (2003) *Integrated Care Records Service: Introduction to the Output Based Specification.* London: NHS.

OECD (1992) *Reform of Health Care: A Comparative Analysis of Seven OECD Countries.* Paris: OECD.

OECD (2005) *Health at a Glance: OECD Indicators 2005.* Paris: OECD.

OECD (2006a) *Factbook 2006 – Economic, Environmental and Social Statistics.* Paris: OECD.

OECD Economics Department (2006b) *Projecting OECD Health and Long-term Care Expenditures: What are the Main Drivers? – Working Paper 477.* Paris: OECD.

OECD (2006c) *OECD Health Data: Statistics and Indicators for 30 countries.* Paris: OECD.

Office of National Statistics (2003) *2001 Census Data – Key statistics.* London: ONS.

Office of National Statistics (2007) *Conceptions in England and Wales 2005.* London: ONS.

O'Connor, J. (1973) *The Fiscal Crisis of the State.* New York: St Martin's Press.

Offe, C. (1984) *Contradictions of the Welfare State.* London: Hutchinson.

Olsen, J. (1983) *Organised Democracy.* Oslo: Universitetsforlaget.

Osborne, T. (1997) 'Of health and statecraft', in Petersen, A. and Bunton, R. (eds). *Foucault, Health and Medicine.* London: Routledge, chapter 9.

Palmer, K. (2006) *NHS Reform : Getting Back on Track.* London: Kings Fund.

Parsons, T. (1951) *The Social System.* New York: Free Press.

Paton, C. (2006) *New Labour's State of Health; Political economy, Public Policy and the NHS.* Aldershot: Ashgate.

Peckham, S., Exworthy, M., Powell, M. and Greener, I. (2006) *Decentralisation, Centralisation and Devolution in Publicly Funded Health Services: Decentralisation as an Organisational model for Health Care in England – A report for the National Co-ordinating Centre for NHS Service Delivery and Organisation Research and Development.* London: NCCDSO.

Petersen, A. (1997) 'Risk, governance and the new public health', in Petersen, A. and Bunton, R. (eds). *Foucault, Health and Medicine.* London: Routledge, chapter 10.

Pierson, C. (1996) *The Modern State.* London: Routledge.

Pierson, P. (2000) 'Not Just What, but When: Timing and Sequence in Political Processes', *Studies in American Political development*, 14: 72–92.

Pocock, S., Collier, T., Dandreo, K., de Stavola, B., Goldman, M., Kalish, L., Kasten, L. and McCormack, V. (2004) 'Issues in the reporting of epidemiological studies: a survey of recent practice', *British Medical Journal*, 329: 883.

Pollitt, C., Girre, X., Lonsdale, J., Mul, R., Summa, H. and Waerness, M. (1999) *Performance or Compliance: Performance Audit and Public Management in Five Countries*. Oxford: Oxford University Press.

Pollock, A. (2004) *NHS plc*. London: Verso.

Powell, M. (1997) *Evaluating the National Health Service*. Buckingham: Open University Press.

Propper, C., Wilson, D. and Burgess, S. (2006) 'Extending choice in English health care: the implications of the economic evidence', *Journal of Social Policy*, 35(4): 537–557.

Putnam, R. (1995) 'Bowling Alone: American's Declining Social Capital', *Journal of Democracy*, 6(1): 65–78.

Ray, L. and Reed, M. (eds) (1994) *Organizing Modernity: New Weberian Perspectives on Work, Organization and Society*. London: Routledge.

Rogers, A., Kennedy, A., Nelson, E. and Robinson, A. (2005) 'Uncovering the Limits of Patient-Centeredness: Implementing a Self-Management Trial for Chronic Illness', *Qualitative Health Research*, 15(2): 224–239.

Royal Pharmaceutical Society (1997) *From Compliance to Concordance: Achieving Shared Goals in Medicine Taking*. London: Royal Pharmaceutical Society.

Sabatier, P. and Mazmanian, D. (1979) 'The conditions of effective implementation: a guide to accomplishing policy objectives', *Policy Analysis*, vol 5: 481–504.

Saltman, R. (2002) 'Regulating incentives: the past and present role of the state in health care systems', *Social Science and Medicine*, Vol 54: 1677–1684.

Saltman, R. (2004a) 'Social health insurance in perspective: the challenge of sustained stability', in Saltman, R., Busse, R. and Figueras, J. (eds). *Social Health Insurance Systems in Western Europe*. Maidenhead: Open University Press. pp. 3–20.

Saltman, R. (2004b) 'Assessing social health insurance systems: present and future policy issues', in Saltman, R., Busse, R. and Figueras, J. (eds). *Social Health Insurance Systems in Western Europe*. Maidenhead: Open University Press. pp. 141–152.

Schmidt, V. (2006) 'Institutionalism', in Hay, C., Lister, M. and Marsh, D. (eds). *The State: Theories and Issues*. Basingstoke: Palgrave Macmillan. pp. 98–117.

Scott, T., Mannion, R., Marshall, M., Davies, H. (2003) 'Does organisational culture influence health care performance? A review of the evidence', *Journal of Health Service Research Policy*, 8(2): 105–117.

Scottish Executive (2000) *Our National Health: A Plan for Action, A Plan for Change*. Edinburgh: Scottish Executive.

Selnick, P. (1985) 'Focusing organisational research on regulation', in Noll, R. (ed). *Regulatory Policy and the Social Sciences*. Berkeley, California: University of California Press.

Shipman Inquiry [chair Dame Janet Smith] (2004) *Safeguarding Patients: Lessons From the Past, Proposals for the Future*. London: Stationery Office.

Simon, H. A. (1957) *Administrative Behaviour* (2nd edn). New York: Macmillan.

Skocpol, T. (1992) *Protecting Soldiers and Mothers*. Cambridge, MA: Harvard University Press.

Sudlow, C. and Counsell, C. (2003) 'Problems with UK government's risk sharing scheme for assessing drugs for multiple sclerosis', *British Medical Journal*, Vol 326: 388–392.

Sutherland Commission (1999) *With Respect to Old Age: Long Term Care – Rights and Responsibilities: a Report by the Royal Commission on Long-term Care*. Cmnd 4192. London: The Stationery Office.

Sutton, M., Gravelle, H., Morris, S., Leyland, A., Windmeijer, F., Dibben, C. and Murihead, M. (2002) *Allocation of Resources to English areas: Individual and Small Area Determinants of Morbidity and the Use of Health Care Resources. Report to the Department of Health*. Edinburgh: Information and Services Division.

Taylor, P. and Donnelly, M. (2006) 'Professional perspectives on decision making about the long-term care of older people', *British Journal of Social Work*, 36: 807–826.

Teenage Pregnancy Unit (2000) *Teenage Pregnancy National Campaign*. London: DoH.

Therborn, G. (1980) *The Ideology of Power and the Power of Ideology*. London: New Left Books.

Timmins, N. (1996) *The Five Giants*. London: Fontana Press.

Titmuss, R. (1958) *Essays on 'The Welfare State'*. London: Unwin University Books.

Titmuss, R. (1968) *Commitment to Welfare*. London: Allen & Unwin.

Titmuss, R. (1970a) *The Gift Relationship: From Human Blood to Social Policy*. London: Allen & Unwin.

Townsend, P. (ed) (1970b) *The Concept of Poverty*. London: Heinemann Educational.

Tudor-Hart, J. (1971) 'The Inverse Care Law', *Lancet*, 27th February: 405–412.

Tudor-Hart, J. (2006) *The Political Economy of Health Care: a Clinical Perspective*. Cambridge: Policy Press.

Tuohy, C. (1999) 'Dynamics of a changing health sphere: the United States, Britain and Canada', *Health Affairs*, 18(3): 114–134.

Tullock, G. (1965) *The Politics of Bureaucracy*. Washington, DC: Public Affairs Press.

Tullock, G. (1976) *The Vote Motive*. London: Institute of Economic Affairs.

Turner, B. (1987) *Medical Power and Social Knowledge*. London: Sage.

Walshe, K. (2003) *Regulating Healthcare: a Prescription for Improvement?* Maidenhead: Open University Press.

Wanless, D. (2001) *Securing our Future Health: Taking a Long-term View – Interim Report*. London: HM Treasury.

Wanless, D. (2002) *Securing our Future Health: Taking a Long-term View – Final Report*. London: HM Treasury.

Wanless, D. (2006) *Securing Good Care for Older People: Taking a Long-term View*. London: King's Fund.

Watson, P. (2004) 'Re-thinking transition: globalism, gender and class', in Scott, J. and Keates, D. (eds). *Going Public: Feminism and the Shifting Boundaries of the Private Sphere*. Urbana and Champaign: University of Illinois Press. pp. 278–308.

Weber, M. (1963) *The Theory of Social and Economic Organisation*. New York: Free Press.

Weber, M. (1978) *Economy and Society* (2 volumes). Berkeley: University of California Press.

Webster, C. (2002) *The National Health Service: A Political History* (2nd edn). Oxford: Oxford University Press.

Whitehead, M. (1998) 'Diffusion of ideas on social inequalities in health: A European perspective', *Milbank Quarterly*, 76(3): 469–492.

Wilkinson, R. (1996) *Unhealthy Societies: the Afflictions of Inequality*. London: Routledge.

Wilsford, D. (1994) 'Path dependency, or why history makes it difficult, but not impossible to reform health systems in a big way', *Journal of Public Policy*, 14(3): 251–283.

Wistow, G. and Hardy, B. (1994) 'Community care planning', in Malin, N. (ed). *Implementing Community Care*. Buckingham: Open University Press. Chap 3.

Wistow, G. and Hardy, B. (1996) 'Competition, Collaboration and Markets', *Journal of Interprofessional Care*, 10(1): 5–10.

Zizěk, S. (1989) *The Sublime Object of Ideology*. London. Verso – Reprinted in Zizek, S. (ed) (1994) *Mapping Ideology*. London: Verso.

INDEX